100 Question R
About Liver
Transplantation:
A Lahey Clinic Guide

Fredric D. Gordon, MD

*Director of Hepatology and Medical Director of
Liver Transplantation
Lahey Clinic Medical Center
Burlington, MA
Assistant Professor of Medicine
Tufts Medical School
Boston, MA*

JONES AND BARTLETT PUBLISHERS
Sudbury, Massachusetts
BOSTON   TORONTO   LONDON   SINGAPORE

World Headquarters

Jones and Bartlett Publishers
40 Tall Pine Drive
Sudbury, MA 01776
978-443-5000
info@jbpub.com
www.jbpub.com

Jones and Bartlett Publishers
Canada
6339 Ormindale Way
Mississauga, Ontario L5V 1J2
CANADA

Jones and Bartlett Publishers
International
Barb House, Barb Mews
London W6 7PA
UK

Jones and Bartlett's books and products are available through most bookstores and online booksellers. To contact Jones and Bartlett Publishers directly, call 800-832-0034, fax 978-443-8000, or visit our website www.jbpub.com.

Substantial discounts on bulk quantities of Jones and Bartlett's publications are available to corporations, professional associations, and other qualified organizations. For details and specific discount information, contact the special sales department at Jones and Bartlett via the above contact information or send an email to specialsales@jbpub.com.

The authors, editor, and publisher have made every effort to provide accurate information. However, they are not responsible for errors, omissions, or for any outcomes related to the use of the contents of this book and take no responsibility for the use of the products described. Treatments and side effects described in this book may not be applicable to all patients; likewise, some patients may require a dose or experience a side effect that is not described herein. The reader should confer with his or her own physician regarding specific treatments and side effects. Drugs and medical devices are discussed that may have limited availability controlled by the Food and Drug Administration (FDA) for use only in a research study or clinical trial. The drug information presented has been derived from reference sources, recently published data, and pharmaceutical research data. Research, clinical practice, and government regulations often change the accepted standard in this field. When consideration is being given to use of any drug in the clinical setting, the health care provider or reader is responsible for determining FDA status of the drug, reading the package insert, reviewing prescribing information for the most up-to-date recommendations on dose, precautions, and contraindications, and determining the appropriate usage for the product. This is especially important in the case of drugs that are new or seldom used.

Production Credits
Executive Publisher: Christopher Davis
Production Director: Amy Rose
Associate Editor: Kathy Richardson
Production Assistant: Jamie Chase
Associate Marketing Manager: Laura Kavigian
Composition: Northeast Compositors, Inc.
Cover Design: Kate Ternullo
Cover Image: © Digital Vision/Getty Images
Cover Image: © Photodisc
Printing and Binding: Malloy
Cover Printing: Malloy

Library of Congress Cataloging-in-Publication Data
Gordon, Fredric D.
    100 questions and answers about liver transplantation : a Lahey Clinic guide / Fredric D. Gordon ; series editor, Andrew S. Warner.
        p. cm.
    Includes bibliographical references and index.
    ISBN-13: 978-0-7637-4048-1
    ISBN-10: 0-7637-4048-9
    1. Liver—Transplantation—Miscellanea. 2. Liver—Transplantation—Popular works. I. Title. II. Title: One hundred questions and answers about liver transplantation.
    RD546.G67 2006
    617.5'5620592—dc22
                                    2006014576
6048

Printed in the United States of America
10 09 08 07 06   10 9 8 7 6 5 4 3 2 1

This book is dedicated to my family—Lynda, Eric, Alyson, and Mandy—
for their never-ending support and patience.

Contents

Introduction   ix

Part 1: The Basics   1

Questions 1–13 cover basic information about the liver and liver disease, including:
- What is the liver, and why is it so important?
- What is cirrhosis?
- I don't drink alcohol and yet I have cirrhosis. How can that be? What causes cirrhosis?

Part 2: Before Transplantation   19

Questions 14–30 address concerns and information prior to transplantation, including:
- Who is a candidate for liver transplantation?
- How do I choose the right liver transplant program?
- What questions should I ask my transplant team to make sure I have chosen the best one for me?

Part 3: Organ Allocation   47

Questions 31–44 look at how organs are allocated, including:
- What is UNOS?
- What is the MELD score?
- How does the waiting list work?

Part 4: Preparing for Transplantation   63

Questions 45–52 look at how to prepare oneself for a transplant, including:
- How do I need to prepare for transplantation?
- How can I best prepare myself physically for transplantation?
- Are there any special diets for people with liver disease?

Part 5: Surgery — 79

Questions 53–57 explore the various factors involving surgery itself, including:
- How long will my liver transplant operation take?
- How will I feel after I wake up from my transplant surgery?
- How long will I be in the hospital?

Part 6: Recurrent Liver Disease — 95

Questions 58–61 address the prospect of liver disease reoccurring after transplantation, including:
- Can my original disease recur in the new liver?
- I was transplanted because of hepatitis C cirrhosis. Will hepatitis C recur in the new liver?
- Is there any treatment for hepatitis C after liver transplantation?

Part 7: Expectations — 103

Questions 62–74 explore what to expect after liver transplantation, including:
- What happens after I am discharged from the hospital?
- Can I drink alcohol after my transplant?
- How long will my liver last after transplantation?

Part 8: Medications — 127

Questions 75–78 address the issue of medication and its side effects, including:
- Why are immunosuppressive drugs necessary?
- What are the immunosuppressive drugs?
- Will I ever be able to stop my immunosuppressive drugs?

Part 9: Complications — 151

Questions 79–84 address possible complications associated with transplantation, including:
- What is acute rejection?
- Now that I am immunosuppressed, am I susceptible to infections?
- What is chronic rejection?

Part 10: Living Donor Liver Transplantation — 161

Questions 85–100 talk about being a donor and prospects for the future, including:
- What is the difference between the right and left lobes of the liver?
- What is a living donor liver transplant?
- What is a split donor liver transplant?

Resources   179

Glossary   183

Index   189

Contents

Since the early 1990s, liver transplantation has become a frequently performed operation for patients with cirrhosis and liver failure. Liver transplantation is performed at over 120 centers in the United States, and more than 5,000 patients undergo liver transplantation each year. While it remains a highly specialized and technically demanding operation, results have improved so much that more than 85 percent of the patients who might have otherwise died are able to survive and return to an active lifestyle. Many of the advances in the field have been technical or pharmaceutical in nature; other advances include improvement in the pre- and post-operative medical care of the recipient. Organ allocation—once a hindrance to fair and equitable access—has now become standardized across the United States, with the patients most in need being placed at the top of the waiting list.

Patient selection for transplantation remains an inexact science. Transplant candidate evaluation and selection are similar at most institutions. The evaluation can be a time-consuming and arduous process for the candidate. This burden can be eased by implementing a strong educational effort about the process, the criteria for acceptance, and the intricate mechanisms of the waiting list. Patients and their families can play an active role in the acquisition of knowledge during the evaluation and waiting time. This helps not only the candidate but also the members of the transplant team caring for the candidate. Knowing what is necessary to be an acceptable candidate can increase the chances of a successful waiting period.

This book is written to give patients with liver disease and their families the tools they need to navigate through the liver transplant system. Many uncertainties persist about the need for transplantation and the requirements of candidacy. *100 Questions & Answers About Liver Transplantation: A Lahey Clinic Guide* demystifies the process so that patients can actively participate in their health care. The book is also useful to people who have already received a liver transplant. It addresses questions related to immunosuppressive medications, long-term success rates and complications, and recurrent liver diseases. This knowledge arms the transplant recipient for the future.

Lastly, *100 Questions & Answers about Liver Transplantation: A Lahey Clinic Guide* addresses the relatively new field of living donor adult liver transplantation. Given the national shortage of donated organs, living donor transplantation may be the only real option for a growing proportion of the candidates on the waiting list. Again, knowledge about the timing of this procedure and the risks and benefits to both the recipient and the donor are critical information.

It is also helpful to hear about real-life experiences with liver transplantation. This book features the voice of Jonathan Kerr as he comments on his life as a liver transplant recipient. Here is Jonathan's story:

At the time of my liver transplant I was a 43-year-old married man with three young daughters. My liver disease had been a part of my life for more than 20 years. I had many flare-ups during this time, but especially in the last 10 years as my health declined. The severity of my illness took its toll on me physically, emotionally, and mentally. When I got to the point where my liver disease had become very serious, a cadaver liver was not an option for me. Time was running out. Out of nowhere, I found myself in a life-or-death situation. It was my younger sister who gave me the "gift of life" on July 26, 2002. Without the healthy lobe of her liver, I would not have survived. Through the tremendous support of my family and friends coupled with the expertise of the liver transplant team, I was given a new lease on life. Words cannot express how I will be forever grateful to all of them, as I can now live a full life as a father, a husband, a son, a brother, an uncle, a teacher, and a friend.

I hope that the information provided in this book educates the reader to be an active participant in the liver transplantation process, whether the transplant is his or her own or that of a loved one.

Fredric D. Gordon, MD

PART ONE

The Basics

What is the liver, and why is it so important?

What is cirrhosis?

I don't drink alcohol and yet I have cirrhosis. How can that be? What causes cirrhosis?

More...

1. What is the liver, and why is it so important?

The **liver** is the largest solid organ in the body. It is located on the right side of the abdomen (to the right of the stomach), behind the lower ribs and below the lungs (Figure 1). The liver is divided into two sections called lobes. In a healthy adult, the liver is about the size of a football, weighing about 2.5 to 3 pounds. This organ receives its blood supply from two sources: the portal vein and the **hepatic** artery. The portal vein brings blood carrying nutrients to the liver from the intestine, and the hepatic artery brings blood and oxygen to the liver from the heart and lungs. The hepatic veins return blood to the heart . The liver performs more than 400 functions each day to keep the body healthy. Some of its major jobs are described here:

- Production of **bile** that permits the body to use protein, fat, and carbohydrates
- Use and storage of fats, sugars, iron, and vitamins
- Production of blood clotting substances such as **prothrombin**
- Detoxification of drugs, alcohol, and other potentially harmful substances
- Production of a protein called albumin, which helps keep the body fluid within the blood vessels
- Monitoring for the presence of **bacteria** in the blood

2. What is cirrhosis?

Cirrhosis means severe scarring of the liver. When normal liver tissue is damaged, it changes into scar tissue or fibrosis. This scar tissue can reduce blood flow through the liver, making it difficult for the liver to

Liver
the largest internal organ of the body; located in the upper right portion of the abdomen. It performs numerous functions vital to life.

Hepatic
having to do with the liver.

The liver performs more than 400 functions each day to keep the body healthy.

Bile
a fluid produced by the liver, stored in the **gallbladder**, and released into the small intestine to help the body digest fats.

Gallbladder
a sac attached to the liver in which bile is stored.

Prothrombin
a substance produced by the liver that helps with clotting. Prothrombin time is a blood test that indirectly measures the ability of the liver to produce prothrombin; it is also known as the international normalized ratio (INR).

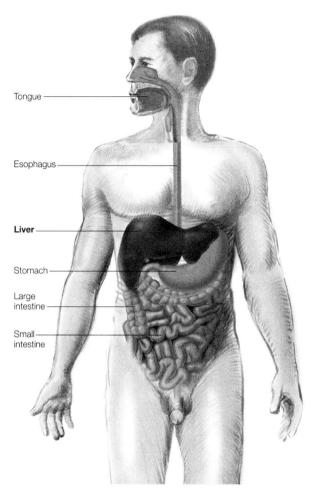

Tongue

Esophagus

Liver

Stomach

Large intestine

Small intestine

Figure 1   Location of the Liver in the Abdomen

carry out functions that are essential for life and health. Many people believe that cirrhosis indicates a history of alcohol abuse, but this is not necessarily true. Many diseases and conditions may potentially cause severe scarring of the liver, including—but not limited to—alcohol abuse. A normal liver has no damage or scar tissue. As damage caused by disease progresses, liver cells die and turn into scar cells.

Many diseases and conditions may potentially cause severe scarring of the liver, including— but not limited to—alcohol abuse.

Bacteria

small organisms or germs that can cause disease.

Cirrhosis

scarring of the liver.

The Basics

3

Jaundice

yellowing of the skin and eyes caused by excess bile products in the blood; a common sign of liver disease.

Cirrhosis rarely causes signs and symptoms in its early stages. When liver function deteriorates, fatigue, exhaustion, nausea, weight loss, and swelling in the legs and abdomen may occur. **Jaundice**—a yellowing of the skin and the whites of the eyes—and intense itching may develop as well.

3. I don't drink alcohol and yet I have cirrhosis. How can that be? What causes cirrhosis?

Virus

a very small germ that causes infection.

Hepatitis

a viral infection or nonspecific inflammation of the liver that can lead to liver failure. Hepatitis C is the leading cause of liver failure that leads to transplantation.

Cirrhosis has many causes (Table 1). Alcohol is one of the most common causes of cirrhosis. It can directly injure healthy liver cells, so that these cells become scar tissue. Alcohol also brings damaging fat into the liver. In the United States, alcohol is not the most common cause of cirrhosis. Fatty liver disease not associated with alcohol use, known as non-alcoholic steatohepatitis, is the leading cause of liver disease in this country. Infection with **viruses** such as **hepatitis** C and hepatitis B can also lead to cirrhosis. In addition, a number of inheritable conditions, such as hereditary hemochromatosis and alpha-1 antitrypsin deficiency, and autoimmune conditions, such as primary biliary cirrhosis and primary sclerosing cholangitis, can lead to cirrhosis.

Jonathan's comments:

In the beginning of my liver disease, the origins were unknown and a mystery. I was eager to figure out the cause. When I got no answers, I had to focus on listening to my body and following the doctor's orders. By the time I was put on the liver transplant list, it no longer mattered how I got sick—my focus was on how I would manage my symptoms and survive.

Table 1 Causes of Cirrhosis
Non-alcoholic steatohepatitis
Hepatitis C
Chronic hepatitis B
Alcoholic liver disease
Primary biliary cirrhosis
Primary sclerosing cholangitis
Hereditary hemochromatosis
Alpha-1 antitrypsin deficiency
Autoimmune hepatitis
Secondary biliary cirrhosis
Budd-Chiari syndrome
Wilson's disease
Congenital hepatic fibrosis
Biliary atresia
Cardiac failure
Cryptogenic cirrhosis

4. What are the complications of cirrhosis?

Many people with cirrhosis have no signs or symptoms at all and feel quite well. In this condition, which is known as *compensated cirrhosis*, even though the liver is severely scarred, there are enough healthy cells within the scar tissue to perform all of the necessary functions of a non-cirrhotic liver. Most people with compensated cirrhosis remain in this condition for life and do not develop further complications of liver disease.

Over time some people with compensated cirrhosis progress to *decompensated cirrhosis*. In this condition, the liver is no longer capable of performing all of its normal functions. Complications that people with decompensated cirrhosis may experience include bleeding varicose veins (**varices**) in the esophagus or stomach, accumulation of fluid in the abdomen (**ascites**), yellowing of the eyes and skin (jaundice),

Most people with compensated cirrhosis remain in this condition for life and do not develop further complications of liver disease.

Varices (esophageal)
enlarged and swollen veins at the bottom of the esophagus, near the stomach. This condition is often caused by increased pressure in the liver, and can cause these veins to ulcerate and bleed.

Ascites
fluid in the abdomen.

The Basics

and confusion due to the liver's inability to clear toxins from the blood (hepatic **encephalopathy** [HE]).

Jonathan's comments:

Because I suffered from decompensated cirrhosis after years of being sick, I struggled at times with edema, some confusion, ascites, and memory loss. It was hard to face the fact that my liver disease had progressed to the point where dramatic changes were occurring. The doctors stressed the importance of listening to those around me if they noticed these changes rather than denying they were indeed happening.

5. What is portal hypertension?

To understand portal hypertension, one must first have a working knowledge of the normal blood flow into and out of the liver (Figure 2). Blood leaves the intestines and flows upward through the mesenteric veins to the portal vein. The blood in these vessels carries all of the nutrients and by-products from digestion of food to the liver. Blood from the spleen also flows toward the portal vein, where it joins the blood from the mesenteric veins. The portal vein carries the blood into the liver, and then splits into right and left branches. These branches then divide over and over again into small capillary vessels. A good analogy for this system is a tree: The tree trunk is the portal vein, and the large branches are the right and left portal veins. The twigs are the capillaries.

A network of vessels also carries blood out of the liver to the heart. These vessels are called the hepatic veins.

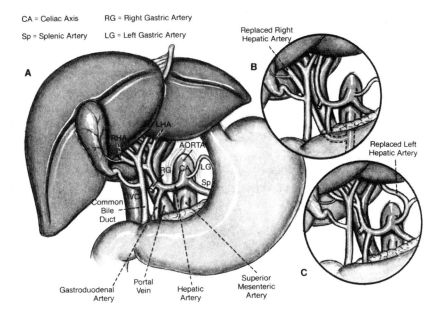

CA = Celiac Axis   RG = Right Gastric Artery

Sp = Splenic Artery   LG = Left Gastric Artery

Replaced Right Hepatic Artery

A

B

Replaced Left Hepatic Artery

LHA

RHA

AORTA

RG CA LG

Sp

Common Bile Duct

VC

C

Gastroduodenal Artery

Portal Vein

Hepatic Artery

Superior Mesenteric Artery

Figure 2   Blood Flow to the Liver. Illustration courtesy of Roger Jenkins, MD, who holds the rights.

To visualize how this system comes together, imagine two trees: one growing out of the ground (the portal venous system) and one hanging upside down from the sky (the hepatic vein system). The trees are connected together by their twigs. Blood flows through the liver by moving up the portal vein, traveling to the right or left branch, continuing on to the portal capillaries (twigs) and then into the hepatic vein capillaries (also twigs), up into the larger hepatic vein branches and ultimately into the inferior vena cava (the trunk of the upside-down tree). From there blood is carried to the heart.

When the liver is damaged due to cirrhosis, the blood finds it difficult to pass from the portal vein system into the hepatic vein system because the capillaries (twigs) are narrowed, twisted, and scarred. Nonetheless, blood continues to flow from the intestinal vessels and spleen toward the portal vein. This results in a "backup" of blood in the portal vein, causing high pressure there. High pressure in the portal vein is also known as portal hypertension.

6. What is variceal bleeding?

One of the most significant complications of cirrhosis is variceal bleeding. It can occur if the pressure in the portal vein becomes elevated (portal hypertension). As mentioned in Question 5, blood enters the liver from the portal vein. When the liver is scarred, the blood flow through the liver can become restricted. Blood is a liquid and will always try to find the path of least resistance. This pathway may be around the liver rather than through the liver. In fact, one of the natural alternative routes circumventing the liver is through the vessels in the esophagus and stomach. These vessels typically carry a small amount of blood at low pressure. When the pressure in these vessels increases, they can rupture, causing a massive hemorrhage and resulting in vomiting of blood and loss of consciousness.

Variceal bleeding is treated with **intravenous** medications, with **endoscopy**, and later with pills called beta blockers. More than 50 percent of patients awaiting liver transplantation will have a variceal bleed prior to transplantation. Frequently, this bleeding is the initial event that prompts the primary **gastroenterologist** to refer the patient to a transplant center. Variceal bleeding is a dramatic event that continues to have a mortality rate of as much as 30 percent despite advances in therapy.

Intravenous

in a vein. Medicines and fluids can be administered through an intravenous line.

Endoscopy

a procedure performed by a gastroenterologist. After the patient is sedated, a long tube containing a miniaturized camera and bright light is advanced through the mouth into the esophagus, stomach, and duodenum. Endoscopy allows the gastroenterologist to view the patient's upper gastrointestinal tract.

Gastroenterologist

a doctor who specializes in the digestive tract and its diseases.

When patients are diagnosed with cirrhosis, endo-scopic evaluation of the esophagus is necessary to assess for the presence of varices. During an endoscopy, the gastroenterologist will administer intravenous sedation. The patient's throat is sprayed with a numbing medication to prevent gagging. An endoscope is then passed through the mouth and into the esophagus, stomach, and duodenum (first part of the small intestine). An endoscope is a long tube with a $\frac{3}{8}$-inch caliber. On the end of the tube are a bright light and a tiny camera. The camera transmits video images to a television screen. Using this system, the gastroenterologist can examine the inside of the esophagus and stomach to determine whether varices are present and, if so, whether they are large or small. If the patient has large varices, then beta blockers can be started to significantly reduce the risk of variceal bleeding.

7. What is ascites, and why does it occur?

Ascites is a complication of portal hypertension and is one of the most difficult complications to manage. As pressure builds in the portal vein, the body tries to reduce this pressure by leeching the liquid part of blood, called plasma, through the vessel walls into the abdomen. Although this transfer of plasma reduces portal pressure, it increases fluid accumulation in the body. The management of ascites requires patience and close attention by both the physician and the patient. The initial treatment of ascites is restriction of dietary **sodium** to less than 2,000 milligrams per day and fluid restriction to 2 liters per day. Diuretics can be added in a progressive, stepwise fashion.

Sodium

an electrolyte that is the main salt in the blood; also one component of table salt.

Occasionally, the fluid accumulation may become so great that the patient experiences pain, limited mobility, and shortness of breath. This problem can be treated with **paracentesis**. Paracentesis is a procedure performed by the gastroenterologist or **hepatologist** in an outpatient setting. An area of the lower abdomen is sterilized with soap and injected with xylocaine (similar to novacaine) to numb it. A needle is inserted through the numb area into the fluid; the fluid is then drained into vacuum bottles or bags. Because this removal of fluid does not actually reduce portal hypertension, the fluid will likely reaccumulate. Frequent paracentesis is not recommended because the detrimental effects increase with more frequent taps. Specifically, essential proteins and nutrients are removed and discarded with each procedure. In patients with chronic liver disease, this often results in severe malnutrition.

8. Why do some people become confused or sleepy when they have cirrhosis?

HE is a frequent but intermittent occurrence in many patients who are awaiting liver transplantation. One of the many jobs of the healthy liver is to clear toxins accumulated from food and metabolism from the bloodstream. When the amount of toxins produced exceeds the liver's ability to clear those toxins from the bloodstream, the person develops HE. This condition results in a temporary change in thought processing. Early signs of HE include insomnia and daytime sleepiness, difficulty concentrating on tasks, and forgetfulness. Later stages are characterized by irritability and other changes in personality, confusion, and sleeping most of the time. HE can even cause coma. This

One of the many jobs of the healthy liver is to clear toxins accumulated from food and metabolism from the bloodstream.

problem usually has an inciting cause, such as gastrointestinal bleeding, poor dietary habits, **electrolyte** abnormalities, **renal failure**, infection, and skipped or excessive medication. In patients presenting with HE, each of these potential causes must be considered and treatment should be directed at reversal of the particular cause.

The initial treatment of HE consists of lactulose. Lactulose is a sweet, syrupy liquid that absorbs toxins and causes diarrhea. It should be dosed so that the patient achieves three to five soft, controllable bowel movements per day. The antibiotics neomycin and rifaximin can be substituted for lactulose or added later if needed.

Many patients with HE are advised to avoid high protein intake. Of all the food types, protein causes much more toxin buildup as compared to fats and carbohydrates. Unfortunately, limiting the intake of protein may result in malnutrition, strength loss, and weight loss, increasing the risk of infection and a poor outcome after transplantation. Protein restriction should be reserved for only patients with HE that cannot be controlled in any other way.

9. What percentage of my liver is functioning?

This is a very difficult question to answer accurately. The function of the liver can be determined by its ability to accomplish its tasks—for example, production of proteins and clotting factors, clearance of toxins, recycling of blood elements such as **bilirubin**, maintaining the **immune system**, and acting as a conduit for blood

Electrolyte
generally refers to the dissolved form of a mineral such as sodium, potassium, magnesium, or chlorine.

Renal
having to do with the kidneys.

Renal failure, acute
when kidneys stop functioning temporarily. Dialysis may be needed until kidney function returns.

Bilirubin
an orange-colored substance in bile that is produced when red blood cells break down.

Immune system
the system that protects the body from foreign substances, such as bacteria, viruses, and cancer cells. It can identify a transplanted organ as foreign and try to eliminate the "invader" from the body.

flow. You do not need every liver cell to be functioning at full capacity for the liver to accomplish these goals. This fact is demonstrated almost every day in hospitals that perform liver surgery. In many of these cases, portions of the liver are removed. After partial resection of the liver, patients may be temporarily left with as little as 50 percent of their original liver size. Nevertheless, during the recovery period, the liver is able to capably complete all of its tasks. Therefore, is it more appropriate to say the liver is functioning at 100 percent or 50 percent (its actual size)? The most important factor is *function* rather than *amount* of liver. It is much easier to think of liver function as "normal," "fair," or "poor" rather than in terms of percentages.

10. What is end-stage liver disease?

End-stage liver disease is an overused and frightening expression. When patients hear this term applied to them, they may fear that they are rapidly approaching poor health and an untimely death. In reality, the origin of this term is much less ominous. Liver biopsies are evaluated for the degree of fibrosis, which is given a score ranging from 1 to 4. Stage 1 means there is a minimal amount of scar tissue in the specimen. Stage 2 implies there is mild scarring. Stage 3 is moderate scarring. Stage 4 fibrosis is equivalent to cirrhosis, which is the last or *end stage*. This designation does not necessarily have end-of-life implications. End-stage liver disease simply means that the patient has cirrhosis. Whether the patient is approaching poor health is better characterized with the terms "compensated" and "decompensated" as discussed earlier.

11. I have cirrhosis. At what point do I need to consider a liver transplant?

The mere presence of cirrhosis is not an indication for liver transplantation. Many people with cirrhosis enjoy normal lives without ever developing complications or the need for hospitalization. Others will decompensate over time, in which case transplantation may become necessary.

Patients often seek out a liver specialist when they first receive a diagnosis of cirrhosis in an effort to learn more about transplantation. Their initial hope may be to have a liver transplant—that is, to remove the damaged organ and replace it with a new, undamaged one. While this outcome might, on the surface, seem to be a good solution, several negative factors must be considered before pursuing this option. First, the rate of surgical complications of liver transplantation may be as high as 15 to 20 percent, including death within the first year after transplantation. You must weigh this risk against the risk of death without transplantation, taking into account quality of life issues. Second, the medications required after transplantation have many side effects. Early exposure to these medications may result in a diminished quality of life for at least some time after the operation. Third, organ availability is limited in many regions of the country. As a consequence, the degree of illness necessary to be at the top of the transplant waiting list can be quite high. Patients with compensated cirrhosis will likely remain at the lower end of the waiting list for a long time.

Many people with cirrhosis enjoy normal lives without ever developing complications or the need for hospitalization.

The Basics

Patients should consider liver transplantation when they have developed complications of liver disease such as ascites, variceal bleeding, hepatic encephalopathy, or jaundice (Table 2). Additionally, even in patients who feel well, a rising Model of End-Stage Liver Disease **(MELD) score** (see Question 32) may be an indication for transplant evaluation. The development of liver cancer my also be an indication for transplantation. Careful monitoring by a physician is necessary in all patients with cirrhosis to look for signs of liver failure so that referral for transplantation occurs at the appropriate time.

MELD score

Model of End-Stage Liver Disease score; the calculation used to rank candidates for liver transplantation. Ranges from 6 (not in need) to 40 (urgent need).

12. Can I become too sick for a liver transplant?

The progression of liver disease is often predictable. Most patients with cirrhosis have already developed complications of liver disease such as ascites, variceal bleeding, jaundice, or encephalopathy. These symptoms may come and go, and the patient may sometimes feel quite well. This is an ideal time for liver transplantation. Unfortunately, because of the system of organ distribution, we rarely have the opportunity to offer liver transplantation at the most opportune time. Livers are

Table 2   Complications of Cirrhosis
Jaundice
Ascites
Variceal bleeding
Hepatic encephalopathy
Malnutrition
Edema
Poor protein production
Poor clotting factor production

distributed according to the MELD scoring system (see Question 32). The MELD scoring system prioritizes patient who are "sicker" based on their laboratory tests (bilirubin, International Normalized Ration [**INR**], and **creatinine**). These lab tests may not, however, reflect the true degree of illness in some people, especially those with ascites, bleeding problems, and malnutrition. This situation may lead to a seesaw of emotions—the desire to rise to the top of the list requires increased illness, but this is a condition no one wishes to achieve.

On rare occasions, candidates for liver transplantation may become "too sick" to undergo transplantation. This situation occurs most commonly when the candidate develops infection or sepsis. In such a case, the infection is often caused by bacteria that enter the urinary **bladder**, **kidneys**, ascites, lungs (pneumonia), or bloodstream. Sepsis can lead to failure of organs other than the liver, such as the kidneys, lungs, heart, and blood vessel (vascular) system. When patients have sepsis, liver transplantation cannot be performed for several reasons:

- **Immunosuppressive agents** are required after transplantation, but they limit the body's ability to assist in fighting off the infection.
- The patient's blood pressure may be too low to safely perform surgery.
- The patient's blood pressure may be too low to adequately supply the new liver with blood.
- If other organs are in failure, a liver transplant may not help the patient achieve total recovery.

In this circumstance, it is better to attempt to control the infection and then proceed to transplanta-

INR

international normalized ratio; a standardized measure of prothrombin time.

Creatinine

a substance that is found in blood and urine. Creatinine is measured to determine kidney function.

Bladder

the part of the urinary tract that receives urine from the kidneys and stores it until urination.

Kidney

one of the two bean-shaped organs located on both sides of the spine, just above the waist. It functions to rid the body of waste and maintain normal amounts of salts, minerals, and fluids through the production of urine.

Immuno-suppressive agents

medicines to control the immune system and prevent rejection of a transplanted organ.

The Basics

tion, rather than the reverse. Unfortunately, when sepsis is present and the liver is not functioning properly, it is difficult for the body to recover adequately to allow later transplantation. It is therefore important to report all signs of infection to your doctor so that early treatment can be initiated and sepsis prevented.

13. Is there any reason to have a liver transplant if I don't have cirrhosis?

Several liver conditions may not progress to cirrhosis yet require liver transplantation. One of these conditions is familial amyloidotic polyneuropathy (FAP). In patients with FAP, the liver produces an abnormal protein, called transthyretin, that can damage the nerves, kidneys, heart, and gastrointestinal tract, but that rarely affects the liver itself. The only way to cure this disease is to replace the liver so that the body produces the normal proteins.

Another non-cirrhotic condition in which liver transplantation is necessary is fulminant hepatic failure (FHF). FHF can be caused by viruses including hepatitis A and hepatitis B, certain drugs such as acetaminophen, rare inherited conditions such as Wilson's disease, and poisons from dangerous mushrooms. In FHF, liver cells become suddenly and severely damaged, resulting in jaundice and encephalopathy. Lifesaving liver transplantation may be necessary in some cases.

Polycystic liver disease (PCLD) results when numerous small and large fluid-filled cysts develop in the liver. The kidneys and **pancreas** can also be affected by

Pancreas

a slender organ located below the stomach and above the intestines. It produces insulin and digestive enzymes.

this disease. Occasionally the liver may become painfully enlarged, limiting the patient's mobility, ability to eat, and comfort, though cirrhosis does not occur. Replacement of the liver will resolve PCLD and will return the patient's abdomen to normal size. Often, transplantation of both a liver and a kidney are necessary if both organs are involved. This type of dual transplant will increase mobility, decrease pain, and improve nutrition. If the patient had been on **dialysis** before transplantation, kidney function will also return to normal and dialysis can stop.

Dialysis

the process by which the blood is cleansed of toxins, and levels of various blood chemicals and fluids are corrected.

The Basics

PART TWO

Before Transplantation

Who is a candidate for liver transplantation?

How do I choose the right liver transplant program?

What questions should I ask my transplant team to make sure I have chosen the best one for me?

More...

14. Who is a candidate for liver transplantation?

If you have cirrhosis with at least some degree of decompensation, you may be a candidate for liver transplantation. To qualify as a candidate for a liver transplant, you must be healthy enough to undergo surgery, be reliable with medication and follow-up appointments, and have a support system at home to help you with your post-transplant program.

Some problems may disqualify you from receiving a liver transplant:

- Alcohol or other substance abuse within at least six months before your consideration for placement on the waiting list
- Metastatic (spreading) malignancy of the liver or other types of cancer
- Other serious diseases, such as uncontrolled infections, uncorrectable heart disease, or severe lung disease
- A history of missing your appointments and poor adherence to or **noncompliance** with prescribed medications
- Inadequate support from family or friends
- **Human immunodeficiency virus (HIV)**-positive status
- A history of multiple upper abdominal surgeries
- Advanced age
- Morbid obesity

If you have cirrhosis with at least some degree of decompensation, you may be a candidate for liver transplantation. To qualify as a candidate for a liver transplant, you must be healthy enough to undergo surgery, be reliable with medication and follow-up appointments, and have a support system at home to help you with your post-transplant program.

Jonathan's comments:

*Being a candidate for a liver transplant requires the **recipient** to make a serious commitment to the aftercare. My younger sister put her life on the line so I could live. I was tremendously motivated to follow all the doctors' orders. This "gift" she gave was a total act of love for me, and [an act of] faith in the liver transplant team.*

15. How do I choose the right liver transplant program?

Choosing the right transplant center is an important decision to be made by the patient and his or her family. You must consider several critical elements when making this decision: the program's success rates, the experience of the team, your proximity to the transplant center, and the degree of collaboration between the medical and surgical physicians in the program.

Program Statistics

The one-year liver **graft survival** and one-year patient survival rates after transplantation are important benchmarks of a program's success. The United Network for Organ Sharing (**UNOS**) publishes these statistics for every transplant program in the nation on its websites (www.unos.org and www.ustransplants.org), allowing you to compare the various programs. If a program's success rates are lower than the national average, it is important to determine the severity of illness of the patients

Noncompliance

failure to follow the instructions of one's healthcare providers, such as not taking medicine as prescribed or not showing up for clinic visits.

Human immunodeficiency virus (HIV)

a virus that destroys cells in the immune system, which makes it difficult for the body to fight off infections, toxins, poisons, and diseases. HIV causes acquired immune deficiency syndrome, a late stage of the viral infection characterized by serious infections, malignancies, and neurologic dysfunctions.

Recipient

the person who receives a donated organ.

Graft survival

when a transplanted tissue or organ is accepted by the body and functions properly. The potential for graft survival increases when the recipient and the donor are closely matched, and when immunosuppressive therapy is used.

UNOS

United Network for Organ Sharing. The private, nonprofit organization that coordinates the U.S. transplant system through the Department of Health and Human Services' Organ Procurement and Transplantation Network contract.

who were transplanted at that specific center before rendering a judgment that program is inadequate. For instance, were the patients older than average or critically ill in the intensive care unit (ICU) prior to the transplant? This information is also available through UNOS.

Experience of the Caregiving Team

Candidates for transplantation must consider the experience of key members of the clinical team. How many transplants has the team performed? Have the team members been together for a long period of time? Do they offer innovative techniques and management strategies? Are they involved in clinical research with the latest treatments?

Proximity to the Transplant Center

During the transplant evaluation, during the waiting period, and after the transplant operation, patients must visit the transplant center frequently. For this reason, you should consider choosing a program close to home to avoid placing an undue burden on you and your support network. Proximity to home may not be the most important issue, however, if there are significant differences in program quality. In addition, your healthcare insurer may cover only certain programs within its network. After weighing all the options, if you find that the best transplant program is not conveniently located, your local physician can collaborate with the program in providing care away from the center.

Coordination of Care

It is important to establish a relationship not only with the surgical transplant team but also with the medical physicians (hepatologists) and nurse coordinators. The medical and nursing teams will play a critical role in your care both before and after the operation. You should be sure that your transplant team integrates the medical, surgical, and nursing components effectively.

In summary, when you are choosing a transplant center, many questions need to be asked and answered. The transplant team members should be accessible, returning phone calls promptly. They should allow you and your family to express their concerns, and they should take the time to address these concerns. The caregiving team should inspire confidence because they work with their transplant patients for many years—before, during, and after the transplant.

16. What questions should I ask my transplant team to make sure I have chosen the best one for me?

You should ask the following questions of a member of the transplant team:

1. Are there any other options besides transplantation?
2. What are the risks and benefits of transplantation?
3. Tell me about the evaluation process?
4. Where is the transplant evaluation performed?
5. How will I know if I am on the transplant waiting list?
6. How long do most patients with my blood type wait for transplantation in this region?
7. How long have this hospital and team been doing liver transplants?
8. Who are the transplant team members?

9. What are the organ and patient survival rates at 1, 3, and 5 years at this hospital?

10. Will I be given an extended criteria donor (ECD) organ? How is that decision made?

11. Does this program offer living donor transplantation? How many of these procedures have been done so far?

12. How many surgeons will be operating on me? How many are attending physicians, fellows, and residents?

13. Is there a special unit in the hospital for transplant recipients?

14. Who can I call with questions about the transplant process?

15. Will I be asked to participate in research studies?

16. Can I tour the transplant center facility and hospital transplant floor?

Jonathan's comments:

When it comes to asking questions prior to having a transplant, my family sat down and thought of all the "what ifs." It is important to feel comfortable asking all of these questions so you can get the answers necessary to relieve some of the anxiety. Once we got the answers, we felt so much more prepared to embark on this medical journey.

17. What is a cadaver liver?

A cadaver liver is an organ obtained from a brain-dead **donor** to be used for liver transplantation. In the unfortunate circumstance of a previously healthy person's death, his or her family may choose to give the

Donor

the person who gives an organ to someone else.

24

"gift of life" and donate the deceased person's organs. Until 1998, **cadavers** were the only adult liver donors in the United States. More recently, organs have been obtained from healthy **living donors**—hence the need to distinguish between cadaveric liver donors and live liver donors.

Most organ donors are people who suffer from head injuries that result in **brain death**. These head injuries may include a stroke, trauma after a car accident or fall, or brain tumor that has not metastasized. Death can be declared in two ways in such cases: when a person's heart stops beating (**cardiac** death) or when the person's brain ceases to function (brain death). Brain death occurs when blood and oxygen cannot flow to the brain, even though the heart is still beating and providing blood and oxygen to other parts of the body. Patients with brain death usually require a **ventilator** or breathing machine to bring oxygen into the lungs. In brain death, the organs remain functional and can be used for transplantation after a physician declares the patient to be brain dead. Because of the potential for conflict of interest, this physician may not be part of a transplant team.

From July 1, 2004, through June 30, 2005, there were 6,082 cadaver donor liver transplants performed in the United States. During the same period, 307 living donor liver transplants took place. While cadaver donors remain the primary source of livers for transplantation, living donation is becoming a feasible option for many patients.

Cadaver

the body of a person who has died.

Living donor

a blood relative or emotionally related friend of the recipient who donates an organ.

Brain death

when the brain has permanently stopped working, as determined by a neurological surgeon, artificial support systems may maintain functions such as heartbeat and respiration for a few days.

Cardiac

having to do with the heart.

Ventilator

a machine that helps a person breathe.

Before Transplantation

18. Who can be a cadaver organ donor?

Anyone up to 85 years of age may be eligible to donate organs and/or tissue. If it becomes appropriate to evaluate someone for organ and/or tissue donation, a trained coordinator will review the person's medical history to determine if he or she can be a donor. People who have died by brain death—that is, cessation of brain function usually due to a traumatic injury or stroke—may be able to donate all of their organs and tissue.

It is important to discuss the issue of organ donation with your family members and your next-of-kin. In most states, merely identifying yourself as an organ donor on your driver's license does not automatically result in organ donation; the surviving family must agree to donation as well. Organ donors are treated the same way as non-organ donors in emergency situations, so you do not have to fear that identification as an organ donor would result in inferior medical care. The donor's body will not be disfigured, so an open-casket funeral can still be an option. There is no charge for being an organ donor.

On rare occasions, a friend or family member of a transplant candidate may die during the waiting period. If the deceased becomes brain dead and his or her family wishes to donate the organs, they may choose directed donation. This means that the donated organs can be directed specifically to the transplant candidate. The Model of End-Stage Liver Disease (MELD) score becomes irrelevant in such a case, and the candidate will receive the liver as long as there is an acceptable blood type and size **match**. The other organs may also be directly donated or go into the standard organ transplant matching system.

Anyone up to 85 years of age may be eligible to donate organs and/or tissue.

Match

the compatibility between a recipient and a donor.

19. What is donation after cardiac death?

Donation after cardiac death (DCD) occurs when there is donation of organs from patients on a ventilator (breathing machine)—usually those with severe brain or nerve injuries, with no hope of meaningful recovery. In ICUs, many techniques for identifying patients with irreversible neurologic injuries have been developed. When it appears that ongoing intensive care is futile, the removal of life-saving measures is often discussed. After consultation with the attending physician, some families make the decision to withdraw ventilatory support to allow their family member to die peacefully. Many of these patients can be organ donors once the heart has stopped beating. After further consultation with an organ bank representative, the family may decide to pursue DCD.

After the decision for DCD has been made, the donor is often brought to or near the operating room. The breathing tube is then removed. Sometimes the family may choose to be present for this step and accompanies the donor to the operating room. If the donor's heart stops beating within 20 minutes, the surgical team, which is already prepared for surgery, quickly removes the donor organs. These organs, which may include the liver, kidneys, and pancreas, can then be transplanted into individuals on the waiting list.

20. What is an extended criteria donor?

To understand the concept of an ECD, one must first define an "ideal" donor. An ideal donor is one for whom there is the expectation of recipient success after liver transplantation. An example is a previously healthy individual, younger than age 40, who is involved in a motor vehicle accident and is immediately evaluated and treated by medical professionals. Despite maximal medical efforts, this patient rapidly progresses to brain death.

An ECD donor differs from an ideal donor in several respects. An ECD donor usually has features that may affect the quality of the liver. For example, the donor may have hepatitis C, be very old, or die after a prolonged illness. The ECD donor may be taking medications to support the blood pressure prior to brain death. The expectation for a successful liver transplant may not be as high as with the ideal donor. Also, the liver graft may take longer to function properly after transplantation, so the recipient may need to remain hospitalized for a longer amount of time than the average organ transplant patient.

Given these limitations, the transplant team must carefully consider whether to use this liver for the top candidate on the list. The shortage of organs in general and especially the shortage of "ideal" organs make the use of ECD livers necessary in many cases. The risk of progression of liver disease and the possibility that an "ideal" organ may never become available are serious considerations when faced with an ECD liver. Many transplant programs have developed specific **criteria** based on research and experience to help make the decision whether to use an ECD liver.

Criteria (medical criteria)
a set of clinical or biologic standards or conditions that must be met.

21. What is a domino liver transplant?

Some people require a liver transplant because they have a hereditary disease called familial amyloidotic polyneuropathy (FAP); FAP prevents the liver from processing certain proteins properly. Although protein processing may be abnormal, the liver from a patient with FAP is normal in all other ways—there is no scar tissue or signs of liver failure. Patients with FAP may develop kidney, heart, gastrointestinal (GI), or nerve problems—all unrelated to their liver disease—usually after the age of 40.

FAP can be corrected by liver transplantation. After a person with FAP receives a new liver, he or she can donate the removed liver to someone on the waiting list. Although the person who receives a liver from a FAP patient will develop the same difficulty processing proteins, this problem is not expected to present until 40 or more years later. In special circumstances, the FAP liver may be split into the left and right lobes, with the different lobes being transplanted into two different recipients from the waiting list. In this way, a single cadaver donor can result in two or three liver transplants.

22. I am the provider in my family and don't usually ask for help. Do I need anyone to help me get through this process?

Liver transplantation requires a major commitment from not only the recipient but also that person's family and support network. An individual often takes many things for granted before becoming ill with liver disease—for example, going to work, driving a car, pushing a grocery cart in the supermarket, and taking medications. After the need for transplantation has been identified, many of these tasks can be difficult to accomplish alone due to weakness, fatigue, and the side effects of medications. Immediately after transplantation, you will not have enough strength or stamina to carry out routine tasks for several months and

Liver transplantation requires a major commitment from not only the recipient but also that person's family and support network.

29

will need help. Your friends and family must be available to drive you to and from your doctors' appointments, to provide food and medications, and to watch for complications of the transplant surgery. You will not likely need 24-hour-a-day nursing care or observation. In fact, you will be able to move freely around your home and gradually go out for short periods of time. Your reliance on others will not last forever; usually, transplant recipients regain their independence in 3 to 6 months.

Jonathan's comments:

When you have a liver transplant, it is vital to look at this medical miracle holistically. By this, I mean you need to pull in all your support systems to get through it. It is important to let others help you in whatever way they can and you need. The transplant affects the whole family, not just the recipient and the donor. Allowing others to help the caregivers and provide moral support and encouragement are vital. The recuperation can be as long as 6 months, which is a long time for any one or two people to support the patient.

23. Should I join a support group?

Joining a support group can be beneficial not only to you but also to your family and friends. Support groups enable you to share your feelings, fears, triumphs, and experiences with other patients in a similar situation as yours. This experience can give you comfort in knowing that your struggles are not unique. Support groups can also give you the confidence and support to continue to battle your liver disease while you are waiting for transplantation. Sharing your emotions with others can provide a release from, and practical advice for dealing with, the stresses of living with chronic liver disease.

Many patients continue to attend their support groups long after they undergo transplantation. It is encouraging to see how the recipients and their families have adjusted to their new lives. Guest speakers are often invited to discuss pre-transplant stress management, advances in surgical techniques and medications, strategies for dealing with insurance companies, and proper nutrition before and after transplantation.

Support comes in a variety of forms—educational programs, group gatherings, social activities, written materials, Internet materials and chat groups, and one-on-one support. Hospital support groups are usually run by the transplant group's social worker or nurse coordinator. They may consist of patients who are waiting for transplantation or those who have already undergone the procedure. Local support groups are usually organized by transplant patients themselves and consist of pre- and post-transplant patients and their families. In these groups, members help other members with practical advice for daily living. Professional organizations, such as the American Liver Foundation, provide seminars, written material, and activities as well. Fundraising to support continuation of their programs and research may also be part of these organizations' activities. Internet support groups encourage you to join a community within the comfort of your own home. They enable you to anonymously ask questions that you may feel are too embarrassing to ask publicly. Be aware, however, that anyone can join an Internet chat group and that the information obtained there may not be entirely accurate or applicable to everyone.

Before Transplantation

24. I have liver disease caused by alcohol. Can I get a liver transplant or do I have to wait in line for a longer time?

Alcoholism is one of the most common causes of liver disease both in the United States and worldwide. Today, alcoholic liver disease is second only to hepatitis C as an indication for transplantation. Many years ago, there were debates about whether patients with liver dysfunction due to alcoholic liver disease qualified for transplantation. Since then, our understanding of alcoholism has evolved; it is now viewed as a disease and, as such, patients suffering from alcoholism receive access equal to that of non-alcoholics in terms of transplants.

The vast majority (more than 90 percent) of the transplant programs in the United States require at least 6 months of total sobriety before transplantation may be considered. The reasoning behind this requirement is neither punishment nor an intentional delay in placement of patients with alcoholic liver disease on the waiting list. Rather, the liver, as a regenerative organ, can improve with abstinence to the point where liver transplantation may no longer be necessary. This process of functional regeneration continues for 1 year or more after stopping alcohol use but is most dramatic during the first 6 months of abstinence. If the patient continues to show signs of liver failure and portal hypertensive complications after 6 months of abstinence, the likelihood of recovery to normal liver function is low and transplantation may be necessary. Most programs also require the patient to undergo rehabilitation and counseling during this 6-month time frame.

The success rates of liver transplantation for alcoholic liver disease are equal to the results for transplantation in cases of non-alcoholic disease. In fact, for those who remain abstinent from alcohol after transplantation, the long-term results may even be better because recurrent disease (such as hepatitis C) is not a concern.

25. What about patients with liver cancer?

Liver cancer is a feared complication of cirrhosis. For patients with cirrhosis on the waiting list, the risk of developing liver cancer can range from 1 to 10 percent. Transplant physicians periodically test the liver for the development of liver cancer by performing an alpha-fetoprotein blood test and conducting an **ultrasound**, computed tomography **(CT) scan**, or magnetic resonance imaging **(MRI)** of the liver.

Some, but not all, patients with liver cancer may be candidates for liver transplantation. To be a viable candidate, the patient must fit into the Milan Criteria (developed at a conference on liver cancer in Milan, Italy). The Milan Criteria state that the patient with liver cancer has a low risk of recurrence after transplantation if

1. There is a single tumor measuring less than 5 centimeters in diameter

   OR

2. There are two or three tumors, each measuring less than 3 centimeters in diameter (Figure 3).

In each case, there must be no evidence that the tumor has spread outside the liver or into blood vessels. A CT or MRI scan of the abdomen and chest as well as a bone scan can rule out spread of the tumor. If there are four tumors in the liver, regardless of their size, the patient is characterized as "outside Milan Criteria."

Ultrasound

a noninvasive radiologic image made using sound waves. It enables clinicians to see and evaluate internal organs and blood vessels.

CT scan

computerized tomography (computerized axial tomography) scan. A noninvasive x-ray that enables clinicians to see and evaluate internal organs and blood vessels.

MRI

magnetic resonance imaging. A noninvasive radiologic image obtained using magnetic energy that enables clinicians to see and evaluate internal organs and blood vessels.

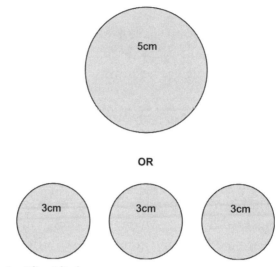

Figure 3   Milan Criteria

In the past, before the Milan Criteria were established and applied, liver transplantation was attempted for a variety of tumor sizes and numbers. When transplantation occurred "outside Milan Criteria," the likelihood of a tumor recurring in the newly transplanted liver was nearly 80 percent within 1 year and nearly 100 percent within 3 years. The reason the tumor is thought to recur in the transplanted liver is related to immunosuppression. The intact immune system has the ability to identify and eradicate any stray tumor cells that may have escaped the liver. Once the liver transplant is performed and the patient begins to take immunosuppressive drugs, however, the immune system may lose its ability to recognize and kill these cells. The tumor cells may then return to the new liver or settle in other sites, such as the lungs or bones. Unfortunately, chemotherapy either before or after transplantation has been largely ineffective in changing the tumor recurrence rates.

Some patients with liver cancer may be candidates for surgical resection of the tumor while awaiting liver transplantation. This procedure may be an option only for patients who have good liver function, minimal ascites, and a tumor located in the left lobe or lower periphery of the right lobe.

26. Who pays for the transplant?

Financial planning is an important part of the transplant process. Each transplant program includes a financial coordinator who will help you understand the cost of transplantation, your insurance transplant benefits, and the overall financial process. You will need to know how much your insurance will pay not only for the transplant itself but also for medications after the transplant takes place. You may find it necessary to draw on savings accounts, investments, federal and private assistance options, and fundraising. The financial coordinator and a social worker can answer questions about insurance coverage and assist you in identifying financial resources available to you.

During your evaluation, you will meet with the social worker and the financial coordinator to discuss financial and social issues in detail. Some insurance companies require a review of your evaluation results to determine whether you meet their criteria before they will agree to pay for a transplant. If you are a good candidate for a transplant, the transplant program will work with you in obtaining insurance approval from your insurance company. Gaining insurance approval is ultimately the patient's responsibility, however.

The cost of transplantation and follow-up varies across the United States. You must consider many potential costs—some directly related to your medical care, others that are unrelated to the surgery. Direct medical care costs include pre-transplant evaluation and testing; surgery and the post-operative hospital stay; subsequent hospital stays for complications; outpatient follow-up care and testing, anti-rejection and other drugs; fees for the hepatologist, surgeon, and anesthesiologist; physical therapy and rehabilitation; and insurance deductibles and co-payments. Indirect costs include transportation to and from the transplant center, food and lodging for your family, child care, and lost wages for you and some family members.

Few patients are able to pay for all of the costs of transplantation from a single income source. Although health insurance companies cover many of the direct costs, savings accounts and other private funds will likely be necessary to pay for other expenses. The transplant social worker and the financial coordinator may be able to suggest alternative sources of funding for those in need, such as charitable organizations, fundraisers, and advocacy groups.

If you *have* insurance coverage:

- Transplants are very expensive, so you should make sure that your healthcare policy does not include any special riders or limitations pertaining to such procedures. Prescription coverage is imperative, as the costs of transplant medications are high. If you have a health maintenance organization or point of service insurance plan, make sure you obtain all necessary referrals to avoid any billing issues.
- If your health plan covers only partial costs, your social worker and/or financial coordinator can help

you find ways to finance the out-of-pocket expenses. There are programs designed to assist transplant recipients with their unique financial needs.

If you *do not have* health insurance coverage:

• Not having health insurance poses a challenge for patients in need of transplants, but your financial coordinator can help you investigate other options, such as state or federal funding and assistance through charitable organizations or advocacy groups.

• Check with your local Medicaid office to see whether you are eligible for this coverage, which is based primarily on income. In addition, most states operate a high-risk health insurance pool for individuals with preexisting conditions who need to purchase an insurance plan. Check with your state's insurance commissioner for more information.

• On the Internet, you can log on to your state's website, where you will find links to government agencies dealing with insurance or health care. You can also consult your local phone book for agency listings under the government section.

• Several agencies will assist you in fundraising, and the social worker and financial coordinator can provide you with information on these resources. If you are out of work due to disability, you should apply for Social Security Disability Insurance. You will become eligible for Medicare coverage after receiving these Social Security benefits for 2 years. For more information, consult the websites for Medicare or the Centers for Medicare and Medicaid Services.

Medicaid

a partnership between the U.S. federal government and the individual states to share the cost of providing medical coverage for recipients of welfare programs. It also allows states to provide the same coverage to low-income workers who are not eligible for welfare. Medicaid programs vary greatly from state to state.

Medicare

the program of the U.S. federal government that provides hospital and medical insurance, through Social Security taxes, to people age 65 and older, those who have permanent kidney failure, and certain people with disabilities.

27. Is there a weight limit for the recipient?

Many liver transplant programs do, indeed, have a weight limit for recipients. Often this limit is based on the body mass index (BMI). The BMI is a calculation that takes into account both the recipient's weight and height:

$$BMI = \frac{\text{Weight in pounds}}{(\text{Height in inches})^2} \times 703$$

A BMI less than 18.5 indicates that the person is underweight. A normal BMI is between 18.5 and 24.9. A BMI more than 25 is considered overweight, and a BMI more than 30 is deemed obese.

The transplant center makes the final decision whether to apply the BMI or any weight limitation. Many programs use a BMI of 35 or 40 as a limit to withhold transplantation. These programs often cite concomitant problems in obese recipients such as heart problems, **diabetes**, sleep apnea, poor wound healing, and long surgical operation times as reasons to delay transplantation. The presence of ascites can influence a person's weight and therefore his or her BMI. Each program has a different way of addressing this issue: Some consider ascites to be part of the overall weight, whereas others subtract the estimated weight attributable to the ascites before calculating the BMI.

Because weight can change, it is important to discuss your BMI with a nutritionist who specializes in liver disease. Sometimes weight reduction by restricting calories is necessary; at other times this measure may be dangerous for the person awaiting

Diabetes

a disease in which people are unable to process sugar in the body correctly.

liver transplantation. The weight attributable to ascites can also be addressed nutritionally by restricting sodium intake and fluid intake. Diuretics can be added if deemed appropriate by the transplant physician.

28. What is a liver transplant evaluation?

People who have a diseased liver may consider transplantation as a treatment option. A transplant evaluation is necessary to determine the risks and benefits of transplantation for each individual, identify potential problems, discuss the options of a living donor transplant, and identify risks for the potential donor.

Much of your transplant-related care will be handled by a transplant hepatologist—a medical physician with expertise in liver disease and management of patients with cirrhosis awaiting liver transplantation. Additional consultation with a **cardiologist** for people with heart disease, a pulmonologist for patients with lung problems, a **nephrologist** for candidates with kidney problems, and an endocrinologist for patients with diabetes may be ordered as needed.

The evaluation for transplantation usually takes place on an outpatient basis but may occur when you are an inpatient in urgent circumstances. During the evaluation you will have a number of medical tests:

- Blood tests to determine your blood type, liver and kidney function, and viruses to which you may have been exposed in the past, such as hepatitis A, B, and C, and HIV
- A chest x-ray to see if your lungs are healthy

A transplant evaluation is necessary to determine the risks and benefits of transplantation for each individual, identify potential problems, discuss the options of a living donor transplant, and identify risks for the potential donor.

Cardiologist

a doctor who specializes in diseases of the heart.

Nephrologist

a doctor who specializes in the kidney and its diseases.

Before Transplantation

- A Doppler ultrasound of the liver, which enables the physician to see your liver and the flow of blood through the arteries and veins
- Tuberculosis testing, called a PPD skin test
- An **electrocardiogram**

Electrocardiogram

a recording of the electrical activity of the heart.

You may also be asked to undergo additional tests such as a colonoscopy, upper endoscopy, echocardiogram, cardiac stress test, and lung function tests.

If you are being evaluated for liver transplantation, you will see a number of healthcare professionals who can assess these issues:

- A transplant surgeon will discuss the operation.
- A social worker will help you identify some of the issues you are facing and talk with you about your ability to handle the responsibilities that come with being a transplant recipient.
- An infectious disease doctor will identify any active or potential issues with infection.
- A psychiatrist, along with the social worker, will help you identify and handle troubling issues such as depression.
- A financial coordinator, along with the social worker, will help you understand insurance issues about liver transplantation.
- A nutritionist will help you plan a diet that will keep you in the best possible health.

You will also meet with a transplant nurse coordinator. The coordinator is an important person in your care—he or she will act as a liaison between you and the other healthcare providers. You can view the coordinator as a resource for information at all points along your path to transplantation.

After your transplant evaluation is complete, the transplant team reviews all of the information gathered in this process. The team may make recommendations for other necessary tests and vaccinations. Ultimately, the team members will decide whether it is the appropriate time to list you for liver transplantation, whether there are outstanding issues that need attention, or whether you are not a candidate for transplantation. A member of the transplant team will see you at a follow-up appointment in the office to discuss this decision and its impact on your future health care.

29. What is hepatorenal syndrome?

Hepatorenal syndrome (HRS) is a condition characterized by worsening kidney function in a patient with severe liver failure. The cause of HRS is unknown, but it is best thought of as an imbalance between substances that increase blood flow and other substances that restrict blood flow to the kidneys. In most instances, the kidney function decreases steadily, either spontaneously or (more commonly) in response to an event such as infection, repeated large-volume paracenteses, or medication toxicity. Patients are rarely admitted to the hospital with diagnosis of HRS; instead, this syndrome is usually caused by some event that occurs in the hospital, such as overly aggressive diuretic therapy, diarrhea, or GI bleeding. Somewhat surprisingly, the kidneys remain capable of normal function in HRS.

The kidney failure is functional rather than structural. Such kidneys have been successfully transplanted and have functioned normally in their new owners. Also, if liver transplantation can be performed early in the course of HRS, kidney function will likely return to normal.

BUN

blood urea nitrogen; a waste product (created when proteins break down) excreted by the kidneys. BUN is tested as an indicator of kidney function.

In the early stages, ascites is usually present in HRS. The presence of the syndrome is suggested by abnormal blood tests—in particular, rising blood urea nitrogren **(BUN)** and creatinine levels. As the syndrome progresses, the individual experiences decreased urine output, usually associated with increasing difficulty in controlling the ascites. The patient becomes drowsy, nauseated, and thirsty. In the final stages of HRS, the patient's blood pressure drops, coma develops, and urine volume falls further. The terminal stages may last a few days to weeks.

HRS must be distinguished from other causes of renal failure. Occasionally, dehydration is the cause of kidney failure. Other conditions that are reversible must be ruled out, including hepatitis B and streptococcal infection.

Treatment of established HRS is difficult. For this reason, healthcare providers emphasize its prevention by avoiding diuretic overdose, treating ascites slowly and recognizing its complications early, and reducing the risks of hemorrhage and infection. Dialysis does not improve survival. A promising new drug, called terlipressin, is currently undergoing extensive research in the United States as a treatment for HRS. Liver transplantation should be considered in such patients, and, if a person receives a transplant early enough in the course of HRS, combination liver/kidney transplantation should not be necessary.

Before Transplantation

30. Is it possible that I will need a liver and kidney transplant?

The kidneys are twin organs located in the back on either side of the spine, protected by the lower ribs. Each kidney is about the size of a fist and weighs about 5 ounces. Although most people have two kidneys, about 1 in every 500 healthy babies is born with just one kidney. You need only one healthy kidney to live normally.

Blood is brought to the kidneys from the heart through large blood vessels called arteries. The kidneys filter the blood as it passes through them, removing wastes and excess salts, minerals, and fluid from the circulation. After it is filtered, the cleansed blood returns to the heart through large blood vessels called veins. From there, the blood circulates throughout the body. By filtering and cleansing the blood, the kidneys maintain the normal amounts of wastes, salts, minerals, and fluid in the body.

Urine is produced from the wastes and fluid removed by your kidneys. The urine formed by each kidney is drained through long, hollow tubes called **ureters** into the bladder, which is located in the lower part of the abdomen. Urine is stored in the bladder until it becomes full. You then feel the urge to urinate. Urination begins when a muscle at the neck of the bladder is relaxed, opening a valve to the urethra. The urethra is a short, hollow tube that drains urine from the bladder out through the opening at the tip of the penis in men or just above the vagina in women.

Ureter

a tube that carries urine from the kidney to the bladder.

The second major function of the kidneys is to produce hormones. These hormones regulate blood pressure, stimulate production of blood in the bone marrow, and help the bones stay strong by increasing the amount of calcium absorbed from food. Hormone production by the kidneys is vital to good health.

If your kidneys do not perform as they should, any of several problems can develop:

Uremia

a toxic condition that results from wastes, such as urea and creatinine, accumulating in the blood.

- If the filtering system of your kidneys fails, wastes, such as urea and excess creatinine, accumulate in your blood (**uremia**).
- If your kidneys do not maintain the correct balance of chemicals and minerals in your blood, an imbalance may occur that can affect the ability of other organs to function properly.
- If your kidneys produce too much of a particular hormone, you may develop high blood pressure.
- If your kidneys produce too little of a particular hormone, you may become anemic (your body does not produce enough red blood cells).

For patients awaiting liver transplantation who develop any of the kidney problems detailed above, combined liver–kidney transplantation may be necessary.

Some patients with liver disease, especially those with cirrhosis, may develop kidney failure as well. This deterioration may be caused by dehydration, infections, and medications such as diuretics and non-steroidal anti-inflammatory drugs like ibuprofen. Kidney function is critical to the liver patient's overall health. This importance is reflected in the MELD score, which is calculated from two liver function tests and the creatinine level (a measure of kidney function). For patients awaiting liver transplantation who develop any of the kidney problems detailed above, combined liver–kidney transplantation may be necessary. In addition, patients with milder forms of kidney dysfunction may need combined organ transplantation because the medications used to prevent **rejection** can be toxic to the kidneys; if the kidneys have only moderate function before transplantation, they will probably be only minimally functional post-transplant.

The need for combined organ transplantation does not, in itself, elevate the patient's ranking on the transplant waiting list. Because the MELD scoring system takes the creatinine level into account, however, patients with kidney failure tend to have high MELD scores and are often at or near the top of the list.

The organs for patients who require combined organ transplantation come from a single **cadaveric donor**. The addition of a kidney transplant to a liver transplant typically adds 1 to 2 hours to the surgery but does not really increase the risk of complications. In a living donor situation, the liver will come from one donor and the kidney from another donor. The operations occur sequentially during the day of surgery— liver first and kidney second.

Rejection

an attempt by the immune system to destroy a transplanted organ because it recognizes the organ to be a foreign, harmful object.

Cadaveric donor

a recently deceased individual whose death does not affect the quality of his or her organs. The individual and his or her family have agreed to donate organs and tissue for transplantation.

Before Transplantation

45

PART THREE

Organ Allocation

What is UNOS?

What is the MELD score?

How does the waiting list work?

More. . .

31. What is UNOS?

The United Network for Organ Sharing (UNOS) is the nonprofit organization that operates the Organ Procurement and Transplantation Network (OPTN) under contract with the U.S. Department of Health and Human Services. In this role UNOS coordinates organ transplant policy development and compliance, maintains the nation's waiting list, matches donated organs with transplant candidates, and collects data on every transplant patient and donor in the United States.

UNOS plays an important role in bringing together the transplant community to protect patients and the public trust by ensuring that organ allocation policies are followed by all transplant centers and organ procurement organizations (OPOs) in the United States. To ensure that life-saving organs are distributed fairly, a number of detailed policies govern the nation's organ transplant system, such as the Model of End-Stage Liver Disease (MELD) scoring system. These policies are developed by reaching a consensus among organ transplant and procurement professionals, patients, and donor families. Adherence to transplant policy is ensured through a comprehensive, systematic auditing and monitoring process. The policy compliance process is designed to maintain the highest standards in patient safety and to foster public trust in the transplant network.

32. What is the MELD score?

MELD was developed in 1994 to assess the risk of a procedure called transjugular intrahepatic portosystemic shunt. Later the MELD score was evaluated as a

Table 3   MELD Scores and Their Mortality Equivalents

MELD Score	Mortality Equivalent
6	1%
22	10%
24	15%
26	20%
29	30%
31	40%
33	50%
35	60%
37	70%
38	80%
40	90%

Organ Allocation

tool to rank patients on the liver transplant waiting list and found to be a fair way to assign cadaveric organs to those most in need of transplantation. The MELD score is actually a question that is answered by a mathematical calculation: "What is the risk of dying with liver disease in the next three months?" (Table 3). In essence, it is a crystal ball with ability to look 3 months into the future. Its accuracy is quite good but, of course, not perfect.

To calculate the MELD score, three laboratory tests are necessary: the total bilirubin level, the international normalized ratio (INR), and the creatinine level. Inserting these laboratory values into the MELD formula yields a score between 6 and 40. As shown in Table 3, a score of 6 indicates that there is a 1 percent chance of dying during the following 3 months and therefore the need for liver transplantation is very small. A MELD score of 40 means there is a 90 per-

The MELD score is actually a question that is answered by a mathematical calculation: "What is the risk of dying with liver disease in the next three months?"

cent chance of death in the next 3 months and transplantation is urgently needed.

The MELD scoring system has been extensively evaluated by the transplant community and is felt to be fair, objective, and unbiased. The MELD score and ranking for liver transplantation do not take into account subjective elements such as quality of life, ability to work, degree of pain, length of time on the waiting list, and number of hospitalizations. In fact, even liver-related complications such as variceal bleeding, ascites, and encephalopathy are not considered in the score. Before the MELD scoring system was approved for ranking candidates on the liver transplant waiting list, it was extensively researched and a computer model was developed based on the experiences of actual patients. The MELD system places all of its emphasis on the candidate's *risk of death* rather than his or her quality of life. Compared to the previous ranking system, MELD is more effective in preventing death before transplantation. Patients are now more likely to have an opportunity to have life-saving transplantation rather than waiting while the less ill undergo transplantation.

Jonathan's comments:

When I found out I was a candidate for a transplant and my health felt out of control, it was reassuring to know there was a system to determine my place in line for a liver transplant.

33. How does the waiting list work?

The liver transplant waiting list is actually four lists, separated by blood type: O, A, B, and AB. Within each list, patients are prioritized by their MELD scores. When a donor liver becomes available, it is matched with the candidate on the waiting list with the highest MELD score in the identical blood group. A person with a MELD score of 29 is ranked ahead of a person with a MELD score of 30. If the donor is a child, the liver will be matched with the highest-ranking pediatric recipient. Although blood type O is considered a universal donor, a blood type O liver is rarely given to a non-O recipient. This situation occurs only when there is a Status 1 patient (see Question 37) in a non-O group and no Status 1 patient on the blood group O list. Also, if a patient with blood group B or AB has a MELD score over 30, he or she is considered for transplantation with an organ from a blood type O donor.

The MELD score can be reassessed as often as the patient's physician feels it is necessary. Any updated information can be used to recalculate and therefore re-rank patients on the waiting list. For patients with a MELD score in the range of 6–10, new MELD scores must be assessed at least once per year. For scores between 10 and 18, updates every 6 months are necessary. For scores between 18 and 24, new lab data are necessary every month. Scores over 24 require weekly updates.

The UNOS system divides the United States into 11 regions (Figure 4). Organs are procured and distributed within each region. For example, a blood type A liver donated in region 1 will go to the highest-ranking candidate on the blood type A list in region 1. Because of this regional procurement and distribution of organs, each region has its own supply and demand for livers. Regions with a high supply of donor organs and a small demand will be able to transplant candidates with lower MELD scores than regions with low sup-

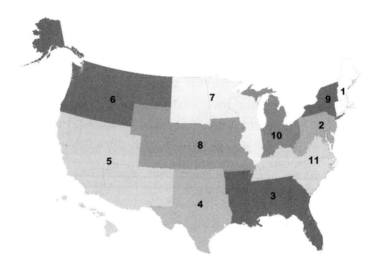

Figure 4   UNOS Map

plies and high demands. This often results in regional inequities in the MELD score needed to appear at the top of the waiting list.

34. What is the Child's score?

The Child's score is an older scoring system used to assess a cirrhotic patient's liver function. It was initially developed by Dr. Child to determine the risk of abdominal (not transplant) surgery. This scoring system has been modified several times over the years to evolve into its current format, the Child-Turcotte-Pugh score. This system assesses five parameters: the total bilirubin level, the prothrombin time, the **albumin** level, the degree of hepatic encephalopathy, and the degree of ascites. Each parameter is given a score between 1 and 3, depending on the severity, and the

Albumin

a protein made by the liver.

scores in the five categories are then added together to produce a total score ranging from 5 to 15. Lower scores indicate better liver health than higher scores. Some physicians group the scores into larger categories. A score of 5 or 6 is called Child's class A, a score of 7–9 is Child's class B, and a score of 10–15 is Child's class C. Presently, to be considered for liver transplantation, the potential recipient must be in Child's class B or C.

35. Is there a national waiting list?

Although UNOS maintains a list of everyone in the United States who is awaiting liver transplantation, there is no functional national waiting list. Because organs are acquired and distributed regionally, the national list does not function on a practical level.

36. Is there anything I can do to move up on the list?

Your position on the waiting list is based exclusively on your MELD score. Movement up (and down) the list is determined by changes in your bilirubin, INR, and creatinine. In the past, the amount of time spent waiting on the list was an important factor in your position on the list. Now waiting time is not considered when determining your rank. For this reason, your doctors may choose to watch you and follow the progression of your liver disease before listing you for transplantation. The transplant team is aware of the typical score required in each region for transplantation and will be able to evaluate and possibly list you as your score approaches the top of the waiting list.

There are presently no limitations on the number and locations of transplant centers you can be evaluated by and listed by. If you and your doctors believe that your condition would benefit from transplantation earlier than might be provided in your home region, you may seek out transplantation in a region that provides organs to patients with lower MELD scores. Unfortunately, there are numerous drawbacks to evaluation and listing outside your home region: fewer readily available family and friend support systems; necessity to travel for evaluation, transplantation, and frequent office visits; and insurance plans that may not cover out-of-region transplantation expenses.

Another option if you seek to undergo transplantation with a low MELD score may be living donor liver transplantation (discussed in Part 10).

37. What is Status 1?

Status 1 is a special designation for patients with fulminant hepatic failure (FHF) and primary graft nonfunction (PGNF). The risk of death from these two conditions is extremely high. Status 1 patients take priority over the MELD scoring system so that these patients can receive the next available liver from an acceptable blood type–matched donor. In this circumstance, patients may receive an identically blood type–matched or a blood type O (universal donor) liver.

FHF occurs when a toxin or virus affects a previously healthy person with a normal liver. Examples include acetaminophen toxicity, mushroom poisoning, and rare instances of hepatitis A or hepatitis B. Affected individuals develop jaundice (yellowing of the eyes and skin) followed within 8 weeks by hepatic encephalopathy (confusion caused by the liver's inability to clear toxins from the blood).

PGNF occurs within 1 week after liver transplantation. Rarely and for unclear reasons, some transplanted livers do not work properly after surgery. PGNF is not caused by rejection or blocked blood vessels. These patients are usually in critical condition and experience liver failure within 48 hours after transplantation; they require immediate retransplantation.

38. What happens if I am not available for transplantation when a liver becomes available for me?

You should alert your transplant team if you are not available while you are active on the waiting list. Status 7 is a designation indicating that the candidate on the waiting list has been temporarily inactivated. Regardless of his or her MELD score, a Status 7 candidate will not receive a liver transplant. Reasons for moving to Status 7 include active infection, sudden hospitalization for an unrelated illness, candidate travel and unavailability, and a change in the support systems necessary for successful recovery from transplantation. Once the issue has been resolved, the candidate can return to active status at his or her MELD score position.

39. Where will my liver come from?

UNOS divides the United States into 11 regions for organ distribution purposes (see Figure 4). Patients waiting for liver transplantation in a specific region will most likely get a liver from their own region, typically from the local **organ procurement organization (OPO)**. An OPO is an organization that is accepted as a member of the OPTN and is authorized by the Centers for Medicare and Medicaid Services to procure organs for transplantation. Each OPO has a defined geographic procurement territory within which the organization concentrates its procurement efforts. A region can have one or more OPOs providing organ procurement services to various locations in the region.

When a cadaveric donor liver becomes available, a standardized protocol is followed to place the organ in the proper candidate on the waiting list. The liver waiting list emphasizes the degree of illness but also incorporates the locations of the donor and the recipient. Status 1 patients have the highest priority for the donor liver first within the local (OPO) territory and then within the region. If there are no Status 1 candidates on the regional list, the liver will go to the candidate with the highest MELD score above 15 within the local area. If no candidates satisfy this criterion, then the liver will stay within the region and go to the person with the highest MELD score above 15. If no candidates in the region have a MELD score greater than 15, then the liver will go to the person with the highest MELD score first in the local area and then in the region. If there are still no appropriate recipients, the liver will be offered to a Status 1 patient outside the donor's region. This system ensures that the sickest local/regional patient has the best opportunity to undergo liver transplantation.

40. Can my new liver give me any illnesses? Is it tested for HIV before I get it?

The organ bank tests donor organs extensively prior to their transplantation. Tests for infection with human immunodeficiency virus (HIV), hepatitis B virus, and hepatitis C virus are performed, and the information is given to the transplant team. Depending on the recipient's disease and severity of illness, the transplant team will have the option of using organs with known infections. Many research papers have shown that placing a donor liver with hepatitis C into a recipient with hepatitis C is safe and does not confer any excess risk of liver failure or severity of recurrent hepatitis C. Similarly, patients with hepatitis B can be transplanted with organs from donors with hepatitis B. HIV-positive organs are not used, however.

Livers are tested not only for viruses but also other infections and conditions that might potentially be passed on to the recipient. For example, a donor with a severe blood infection with the *Staphylococcus* bacteria would not be considered a safe donor because the bacterial infection would likely be transmitted to the recipient. Even if the recipient is currently taking preventive antibiotics, he or she will soon be immunosuppressed; as a consequence, the risk of overwhelming infection immediately after transplantation is very high. The liver and other abdominal organs are also inspected for the presence of non-liver-related cancer.

Organ banks are also adept at acquiring historical information about the donor. Important factors in determining the donor's eligibility include the donor's history of drug use, sexual contact, home situation, nutrition, and prior cancers such as melanoma, basal cell skin cancer, and breast cancer. These considerations are risk factors for the potential presence of infectious diseases and communicable malignancies. This information, when provided to the recipient's transplant team, can be used in making the decision whether to accept that particular organ for the recipient.

41. Can I be evaluated and listed at more than one program? Do I have to move there?

Liver transplantation candidates can be listed at more than one center at any given time, but will not benefit from being listed by two programs within the same organ allocation region. All transplant programs within a UNOS region work from the same master list.

If a patient chooses to be listed by two programs, he or she should be evaluated in different UNOS regions to minimize the waiting time. It is not a UNOS requirement that patients move their homes to the transplant center's region. However, you must consider some additional issues when seeking a multiple listing. First, your health insurance company may not pay for a transplant at a center outside of your local region. Second, if the insurer does agree to pay for the transplant wherever it occurs first, the payer often will not cover the expenses of transportation and accommodation for you and your family. Third, organs become available on very short notice, and you must be able to get to the transplant center quickly once the organ is ready.

Fourth, most programs require their recipients to remain in close proximity to the transplant center for a month or more following the operation to monitor the recovery, watch for rejection, and adjust medications as needed. Finally, if serious post-transplant complications arise, you must be prepared to return to the transplant center for care. These requirements can be very expensive and time-consuming for both patient and family. Even though the waiting time may be shorter at a particular center outside of your home region, it may not be the best overall plan to be transplanted there.

42. Will I receive a liver from a person of the opposite sex?

You may receive a liver from a donor of the opposite sex. As long as the donor liver has a matching blood type, is of adequate size, and is free from transmittable diseases, it can be used for a recipient of either gender. Some data suggest that transplants of female donor livers into male recipients have a slightly worse outcome compared to all other matching possibilities. Nonetheless, even in this situation, the small risk of this outcome does not warrant skipping an offer for a liver transplant to await a male donor for a male recipient. There is no possibility of taking on the characteristics of the donor even in a gender-mismatched pair.

43. What are the acceptable blood type matches for people on the waiting list?

The cadaver transplant waiting list is arranged by blood group. In general, candidates on the list will receive an identically blood group–matched liver (as determined by **ABO typing**) without regard to Rh

ABO typing
a blood test to determine blood type. A transplant donor and a recipient must have compatible blood types.

Table 4   Acceptable Matches of Recipient and Donor Blood Types

Recipient Blood Type	Donor Blood Type
O	O
A	O, A
B	O, B
AB	O, A, B, AB

factor (Rhesus factor, the + or − sign that occurs after the blood type). Fortunately, matching the Rh factor does not seem to have a positive or negative influence on the outcome of the transplant or on rejection. This enables more livers to be used in more transplant candidates on the list. Thus blood type O livers will go into blood type O recipients; A livers into A recipients; B livers into B recipients; and AB livers into AB recipients (Table 4).

Because most people have blood type A or O, these groups tend to have the longest waiting lists but frequent opportunities for liver transplantation because there will also be more A or O donors. Blood groups B and AB tend to have shorter waiting lists; however, because there are fewer people with these blood groups, there will be fewer matching donors. On average, the different blood groups all have relatively equal access to donors within the same time frame.

Only in the rare circumstance of a Status 1 patient or a candidate with blood type B or AB and a MELD score over 25 might a blood type O liver be used in a non-blood type O recipient. Blood type O is the universal donor type, meaning that it can be safely used in all other blood type recipients. The regular practice of using blood type O donors for any other blood group would disadvantage the blood type O candidates on the waiting list, so this practice is not permitted except in emergency circumstances.

When living donor liver transplantation is considered, any acceptable blood group match would be considered. For example, a donor with blood type O can donate his or her liver to a recipient with any blood type. Similarly, a recipient with blood type AB (the universal recipient) can accept a liver from a donor with any blood type.

44. I've just been listed for liver transplantation. How long will it take until I get transplanted?

There is no way to predict just how long it will take until you move to the top of the transplant waiting list. Because the list is organized by blood group and MELD score, waiting time is no longer relevant in distributing donor organs. Until February 2002, when the MELD scoring system was implemented, waiting time was a critical factor in getting to the top of the list. Simply put, the longer you were on the list, the higher on the list you were placed. The list worked very much like a line to buy movie tickets: If you waited long enough, eventually you got to the ticket window. Because this system allowed people who were not in desperate need to undergo transplantation while terribly ill patients died without the opportunity to receive a donor organ, it was abandoned. Additionally, the candidate's location on the list depended more on when the referring physician decided to send the patient to the transplant program than on the patient's actual degree of illness.

The MELD system is based exclusively on the degree of illness and risk of death before transplantation. Waiting time cannot be predicted because receipt of an organ requires a deterioration in health and especially in the three critical lab tests: total bilirubin, INR, and creatinine. Primary care physicians, gastroenterologists, and transplant physicians work diligently with their patients to keep them healthy. The goal is to keep patients well enough so that transplantation is a last resort.

The MELD system is based exclusively on the degree of illness and risk of death before transplantation. Waiting time cannot be predicted because receipt of an organ requires a deterioration in health and especially in the three critical lab tests: total bilirubin, INR, and creatinine.

Certain UNOS regions in the United States have larger supplies and fewer demands for livers than other regions. The result: variations in waiting times across the country. When the demand is high and the supply of donor livers is low, a person must have a higher MELD score to appear at the top of the list. The score needed to undergo transplantation in such regions is often in the range of 30–35. Other regions have large numbers of liver donors, so transplantation can occur at lower MELD scores in the 18–20 range. The reasons for the regional differences in donation rates are not clear but may include differences in fatality rates from motor vehicle crashes, access to major hospitals, regional customs and beliefs, and expertise of organ banks in recruiting donors.

PART FOUR

Preparing for Transplantation

How do I need to prepare for transplantation?

How can I best prepare myself physically
for transplantation?

Are there any special diets for people with
liver disease?

More . . .

45. How do I need to prepare for transplantation?

If you have an active status on the transplant waiting list, it is important that your transplant team be able to contact you day and night, no matter where you are. There is a limited amount of time (60 minutes) during which the transplant team must decide whether to accept or decline an offer of a donor liver. If you cannot be contacted, the team will pass the liver on to the next candidate. Your transplant team may provide or suggest that you purchase a beeper. Make a list of people who need to be notified that you are having a liver transplant. Have someone make these calls while you are on the way to the hospital.

You may wish to consider packing an overnight bag in preparation for your hospitalization. You can include personal items, a bathrobe, slippers, and other items to make your stay more comfortable. You should leave valuables at home, however. You may need a phone card, credit card, or cell phone to make personal calls. Of course, you probably will not have to rush emergently to the hospital once you are called. Instead, you will likely have several hours to arrive—but packing a bag will be one less concern if you have already taken this step. If you are driving to the hospital, choose someone to drive you who will be available when the time comes. You may also wish to designate a backup driver. Become familiar with the route to the hospital and where you will need to go when you arrive. If you will be flying to the hospital, gather information on the flight schedules of several airlines and alternative travel options. You will also need a plan to get from the airport to the hospital.

If you have children, plan who will take care of them during your hospitalization. They may even need care plans that can begin in the middle of the night. If they are old enough to understand, talk to your children about your need for surgery and explain that you will be away from home during your hospitalization. Keep them abreast of the plans for their care while you are away.

It is important to establish a healthcare proxy, living will, or power of attorney prior to undergoing the transplantation procedure. Although the expectation with transplantation is rapid success, you may be incapacitated and unable to make decisions on your own behalf at some point. Discuss your wishes with your family or healthcare proxy so that these parties are fully informed and can carry out your plan. Your physician or social worker can help you with this difficult task.

Lastly, take steps to ensure that you are in the best possible health prior to your surgery. Eat a healthy diet, take your medications, exercise, and talk about your feelings. Spend time with your family and friends, and avoid stress as much as possible.

Jonathan's comments:

As the father of three young children, it was difficult on so many levels to be in such a critical place with my health. My wife and I made a conscious decision to screen the kids from scary information and provide them with a healthy balance of age-appropriate facts. They knew I was very sick and the doctors were going to do everything they could to make me better. During the actual hospitalization, the girls were with a family member they felt totally comfortable with and had regular contact with my wife. We did not allow our children to come and visit until I was stable after the transplant. They asked all sorts of questions and I answered them honestly, though sparing them of details

Take steps to ensure that you are in the best possible health prior to your surgery.

that might frighten them. After my hospitalization, the kids were my inspiration. Their gentleness and compassion fed my spirit and helped me heal.

46. How can I best prepare myself physically for transplantation?

While you are waiting for your transplant, you should try to remain as physically fit as possible. This will aid in your recovery. Even if you become weak and unable to leave your home, you can still exercise to some degree. Deep breathing, tightening and relaxing your muscles, stretching, and leg lifts are possible. You can try to do some light weightlifting with soup cans or rolls of coins. Walking is an excellent form of aerobic exercise that will help you maintain fitness and stamina.

It is important to be realistic about your goals. The longer you have been ill, the longer it will take you to regain your strength. This applies to both the patient awaiting transplantation and the recipient of a transplanted organ. You may want to seek out the assistance of a physical therapist to set up a reasonable program with achievable goals. Your body will tell you when you are overdoing things. If you feel pain or excessive fatigue, you may have done too much and should rest. Even though the level of exercise may be light, it is important to warm up in the beginning and to cool down at the end. Stay well hydrated, albeit within the limits your doctor has recommended if you have fluid retention problems. You must realize that you will have "good" days and "bad" days, and you should adjust your workout accordingly.

You may wish to join a local health club or community center. Exercising with others can be motivational and keep you on a regular schedule. Try to schedule your exercise during your "best" time of day. For some people, this will be early in the day; for others, exercising later is better. Also, try to vary your workouts to keep them interesting. Your level of fitness will have a direct correlation with your recovery after transplantation.

47. Are there any special diets for people with liver disease?

In many diseases, adhering to a specific diet is helpful in controlling the progression of the disease. For example, patients with heart disease can reduce the risk of heart attack by following a low-fat, low-**cholesterol** diet. Unfortunately, no specific diets appear to benefit the liver directly. Instead, you should focus on eating a generally healthy diet with the recommended balance of food groups. Eating a healthy amount of fruits, vegetables, cereals, and meat will provide you with the proper balance of carbohydrates, fats, and proteins. Some patients with liver disease have diminished appetites and require supplementation with small-volume, high-calorie, well-balanced liquid meals such as Ensure, Boost, and Sustecal. Eating more-frequent, smaller meals may be helpful as well.

Many patients with liver disease are prescribed dietary modifications to help them manage some of the side effects of cirrhosis. For example, patients with fluid retention (ascites or **edema**) should be on a low-sodium (approximately 2,000 milligrams per day) and fluid-restricted (approximately 2 liters or 67 ounces per

Cholesterol

a form of fat that the body needs to perform certain functions. Too much cholesterol can cause heart disease.

Edema

excess fluid in the tissues of the body. Swollen ankles are a sign of edema.

day) diet. A dietitian from the liver transplant team can give you practical advice on how to meet these goals.

Patients with hepatic encephalopathy are often advised to significantly reduce their protein intake so as to gain better control of their encephalopathy. This recommendation can be dangerous and may result in severe protein malnutrition, which in turn may lead to muscle wasting, weakness, and poor wound healing. While it is true that proteins are metabolized into more of the toxins responsible for hepatic encephalopathy compared to other food types, proteins are a necessary part of the diet. Patients with advanced liver disease are catabolic—that is, they are not adding fat and muscle to their bodies. Instead, the calories and energy brought in by their food intake are used to address the needs of the liver and other organs. In fact, these patients need *more* calories and proteins than healthy individuals just to maintain their weight and muscle mass. Thus any limitation of protein results in progressive loss of muscle and body weight.

Vitamin supplementation may also be necessary, particularly in patients with the cholestatic liver diseases of primary biliary cirrhosis and primary sclerosing cholangitis. These patients may become deficient in vitamins A, D, E, and K. If patients with liver disease can eat a healthy diet, then adding the standard multivitamins to the diet is usually not necessary.

48. I've been advised to have a TIPS procedure. What is this, and will it help me get a liver transplant?

TIPS stands for Transjugular Intrahepatic Portosystemic Shunt. A TIPS procedure is undertaken to treat some of the complications of portal hypertension, particularly variceal bleeding and ascites. For patients with variceal bleeding that cannot be controlled with medication and endoscopy, TIPS may be a good alternative. Similarly, for patients with ascites who require frequent large-volume paracenteses, TIPS may decrease the need for this procedure and increase the effectiveness of fluid management measures.

A TIPS is placed by a radiologist while the patient is under general anesthesia or conscious sedation. A small catheter is placed in the jugular vein on the right side of the neck (*transjugular*). A flexible wire is advanced through the catheter to the hepatic veins. The tip of the wire includes a retractable needle, which is used to burrow through the liver tissue (*intrahepatic*) until the portal vein is identified. The needle is then retracted. A deflated oblong balloon is then advanced over the wire and positioned between the hepatic vein and the portal vein. The balloon is inflated, creating a track between the portal vein and hepatic vein system (*portosystemic*). The balloon is removed, and a metal mesh tube is advanced over the wire to bridge (*shunt*) the portal vein with the hepatic vein. In this way, a "new" blood vessel is built within the liver. After a TIPS procedure, blood can flow either in the normal direction through the liver or through the TIPS. The availability of the alternative path lowers the portal pressure, resulting in less production of ascites and decreased pressure in the varices.

A TIPS procedure can be thought of as a "bridge to transplantation." It does not improve the function of the liver or have a direct effect on a patient's Model of End-Stage Liver Disease (MELD) score or standing on the transplant waiting list. Rather, it helps the patient and the physician deal with two complications of portal hypertension. Unfortunately, a TIPS can worsen a third complication of portal hypertension: hepatic encephalopathy. The blood flowing through the TIPS does not come in contact with the liver cells that are responsible for removing toxins and by-products from the bloodstream. Thus toxin-rich blood reaches the heart and circulates throughout the body, causing encephalopathy. Nonetheless, TIPS can be helpful for patients who are waiting for liver transplantation by reducing the number of complications and hospitalizations they experience.

49. I've heard that Tylenol is dangerous for the liver. Is this true, and are there any medications I need to avoid?

Oral

by mouth. Many medicines are taken orally in liquid or pill form.

Almost all **oral** medications are absorbed into the bloodstream and carried immediately to the liver for processing. It is therefore important to avoid medications that can cause liver damage. Most prescription medications are safe for the liver, although some require a reduction in dose for patients with liver disease. If you have any questions about the safety of a new medication you have been prescribed, you should discuss your concerns with the prescribing physician and/or a member of the transplant team. Several commonly prescribed medications are worthy of specific mention in conjunction with liver disease.

Acetaminophen (Tylenol). Acetaminophen is a medication that is available in both prescription strength and as an over-the-counter drug. Acetaminophen is commonly combined with other pain medications such as oxycodone (Percocet), hydromorphone (Vicodin), and propoxyphene (Darvocet). It is also found in many flu, cold, and headache preparations. Contrary to popular belief, acetaminophen can be taken safely by patients with liver disease, as long as they adhere to some limitations.

When swallowed, acetaminophen is absorbed into the blood and normally broken down into two parts: the part that controls flu and headache symptoms and a substance that is toxic to the liver. Fortunately, a detoxifier, called glutathione, is waiting for the toxin to arrive in the liver. Glutathione is rapidly, but not instantaneously, reproduced by the liver. The damaged liver may have a slower rate of glutathione production but nonetheless has a replenishable supply. Acetaminophen in doses up to 2,000 milligrams per 24 hours can be effectively detoxified even by the cirrhotic liver. It is important to note that acetaminophen does not slowly damage the liver and that it cannot cause cirrhosis. Because acetaminophen is found in many common medications, you should recognize that the total daily dose may come from different sources of acetaminophen.

Cholesterol-Lowering Agents. Cholesterol control has improved dramatically since the introduction of the cholesterol-lowering agents known as statins. One of the side effects of this class of drugs is liver cell toxicity, although this problem occurs in only a minority of patients. For patients with liver disease, these drugs can be used with caution. First, however, you should determine whether a reduction in your cholesterol level is required. Lowering your cholesterol level reduces your risk of stroke and heart attack over the course of many years. For most patients with advanced liver disease, this may not be a priority, so use of the statins can be avoided until after transplantation. Other patients may have a strong family history of coronary artery disease and stroke or may have had a heart attack themselves; in this group, the statins may be necessary therapy. If a potentially liver-toxic drug is deemed to be of benefit to a particular patient, levels of the **liver enzymes** can be followed closely to confirm that liver toxicity is not occurring. These tests should be performed several times over the first 3 months of prescription use and then periodically thereafter. If the enzyme levels rise above the baseline and remain high, the medication should be stopped.

Psychiatric Medications. Like the cholesterol-lowering agents, many psychiatric medications—but particularly the older ones—have the potential to cause liver damage. This effect occurs only rarely with use of the newer selective serotonin reuptake inhibitors such as Prozac, Paxil, and Celexa. Again, if a potentially liver-toxic drug is deemed to be of benefit to a particular patient, the liver enzyme levels can be followed closely to rule out liver toxicity. These tests should be performed several times over the first 3 months of prescription use and then periodically thereafter. If the enzyme levels rise above the baseline and remain high, the medication should be stopped.

50. Can I take nontraditional medications, such as Chinese herbs?

Many alternative medicinal therapies that are available without prescription are touted as cures for liver disease, "liver health enhancers," or "liver cleansers." None of these supplements has been proven to be effective or, for that matter, ineffective. Few, if any, sci-

Liver enzymes (SGOT/AST and SGPT/ALT) substances produced by the liver. When the liver suffers an injury, these enzymes are produced in large amounts and can be measured in the blood.

entific studies have evaluated the safety and efficacy of these nontraditional treatments. Also, the potential for interactions with other prescribed medications has not been defined for all herbal remedies. Because these substances are not controlled by the U.S. Food and Drug Administration (FDA), their packaging may not reflect the actual contents of the pill bottle.

In general, it is probably best to avoid these medications before transplantation. After transplantation, they should not be taken at all, because the interactions with the critically important immunosuppressive agents are unknown. An interaction with an immuno-suppressive agent may result in inactivation of the pre-scribed drug, which in turn may lead to rejection of the transplanted organ. Alternatively, the herb may increase the blood levels of the immunosuppressant, leading to toxic levels of the drug.

Because the brand names of products vary widely, you should always read labels carefully and look for the following supplement ingredients.

Definitely Hazardous

- **Aristolochic acid** (Aristolochia, birthwort, snake-root, snakeweed, snagree root, sangrel, serpentary, wild ginger): Listed as causing human cancers and kidney failure.

Very Likely Hazardous

These substances are banned in other countries, have an FDA warning in the United States, or show adverse effects in studies.

- **Comfrey** (Symphytum officinale, ass ear, black root, blackwort, bruisewort, consolidae radix, consound, gum plant, healing herb, knitback, knitbone, salsify, slippery root, symphytum radix, wallwort): Abnormal liver function or damage, often irreversible; deaths reported.
- **Androstenedione** (4-androstene-3, 17-dione, andro, androstene): Increased cancer risks and decreases in "good" HDL cholesterol have been reported.
- **Chaparral** (Larrea divaricata, creosote bush, greasewood, hediondilla, jarilla, larreastat): Abnormal liver function has been linked to its use.
- **Germander** (Teucrium chamaedrys, wall germander, wild germander): Abnormal liver function has been linked to its use.
- **Kava** (Piper methysticum, ava, awa, gea, gi, intoxicating pepper, kao, kavain, kawa-pfeffer, kew, long pepper, malohu, maluk, meruk, milik, rauschpfeffer, sakau, tonga, wurzelstock, yagona, yangona): Abnormal liver function has been linked to its use.

Likely Hazardous

These substances have been associated with adverse-event reports or theoretical risks.

- **Bitter orange** (Citrus aurantium, green orange, kijitsu, neroli oil, Seville orange, shangzhou zhiqiao, sour orange, zhi oiao, zhi xhi): High blood pressure; increased risk of heart arrhythmias, heart attack, and stroke.
- **Organ/glandular extracts** (brain/adrenal/pituitary/placenta/other gland "substance" or "concentrate"):

Theoretical risk of mad cow disease, particularly from brain extracts.

- **Lobelia** (Lobelia inflata, asthma weed, bladderpod, emetic herb, gagroot, lobelie, Indian tobacco, puke-weed, vomit wort, wild tobacco): Difficulty breathing and rapid heart rate.
- **Pennyroyal oil** (Hedeoma pulegioides, lurk-in-the-ditch, mosquito plant, piliolerial, pudding grass, pulegium, run-by-the-ground, squaw balm, squawmint, stinking balm, tickweed): Liver and kidney failure, nerve damage, convulsions, abdominal tenderness, burning of the throat are risks; deaths have been reported.
- **Scullcap** (Scutellaria lateriflora, blue pimpernel, helmet flower, hoodwort, mad weed, mad-dog herb, mad-dog weed, quaker bonnet, scutelluria, skull-cap): Liver damage.
- **Yohimbe** (Pausinystalia yohimbe, johimbi, yohim-behe, yohimbine): Blood pressure changes, heart-beat irregularities, and heart attacks have been reported.

It is important to tell your doctor about any dietary supplement you may be taking.

51. My MELD score is low, but I have been diagnosed with liver cancer. How can I get a liver transplant before the cancer spreads?

Many patients with liver cancer have normally functioning livers. Although the risk of liver cancer is significantly increased in patients with cirrhosis, liver cancer does not mean that the liver has failed or decompensated. As a consequence, many people with liver cancer have low (or good) MELD scores. A low MELD score places a candidate near the bottom of the liver transplant waiting list. Despite this low ranking, a liver transplant is needed before the tumor spreads or grows in size or number such that it is no longer within the Milan Criteria (see Question 25).

The United Network for Organ Sharing has recognized the potential difficulty for liver cancer patients in rising to the top of the waiting list based on their calculated MELD score. The solution currently in place is the awarding of a set number of MELD points regardless of the calculated MELD score for patients with liver cancer. Patients with hepatocellular carcinoma (liver cancer) larger than 1.9 centimeters and within the Milan Criteria automatically receive 20 MELD points. If liver transplantation has not occurred within the following 3 months, then a repeat computed tomography scan or magnetic resonance image of the liver is performed. If the cancer is still within the Milan Criteria, the MELD score is reassigned to 24. Again, if no transplant has been performed over the next 3 months and the patient remains within the Milan Criteria, the MELD score is adjusted to 28. Every 3 months, the MELD score is allowed to increase until the patient receives a transplant. In this way, patients with the combination of a normally functioning liver and hepatocellular carcinoma are given a fair chance to undergo transplantation.

52. How long do I have to get to the hospital once I am called?

In most cases, patients called in from home for a liver transplant will have 4 to 6 hours to arrive at the hospital.

Occasionally, the operation may need to occur more quickly. The surgeon will let you know the necessary arrival time. If you cannot arrive in the necessary time frame, the liver will be offered to the next person on the waiting list. You will not lose your position on the list and may be offered the next available organ if your MELD score remains high.

Typically, the transplant team will be notified that there is a potential donor at another hospital late in the day. Often the procurement operation (the surgical team removing the donated organs from the donor) occurs at night. Depending on the distance from the transplant center, the recipient may be notified in the late evening and asked to arrive around midnight while the organs are being procured. Most liver transplant surgeries begin in the morning. Occasionally (perhaps 25 percent of the time), the procured organ is deemed unacceptable for transplantation and the recipient is sent home from the hospital to await another donor. The recipient does not move forward or backward on the list if this occurs.

PART FIVE

Surgery

How long will my liver transplant operation take?

How will I feel after I wake up from
my transplant surgery?

How long will I be in the hospital?

More...

53. How long will my liver transplant operation take?

Liver transplant surgery can take as little time as 4 hours or as long as 12 to 15 hours. Many factors determine the length of the operation, including the experience of the surgical transplant team, the number of surgeries the recipient has undergone in the past, and the degree of the recipient's illness.

In the preoperative holding area, you will meet the anesthesiologist who will care for you during your operation, and you will sign a consent form to permit him or her to give you **anesthesia** for the operation. A lot of activity will occur in this area as the medical staff prepares you for the surgery. Intravenous (in the vein) and arterial (in the artery) lines will be placed in your arm and neck. These lines will still be in place when you wake up after the surgery. Electrocardiogram leads will be placed on your chest to monitor your heart as well. All of these preparations are needed to perform the transplant operation safely. When these preparations are complete, you will be wheeled into the operating room on a stretcher for your transplant operation.

Anesthesia

medicine that is given by a specially trained physician or nurse to put a patient to sleep (general anesthesia) or numb an area of the body (local anesthesia) so that a medical procedure or operation can be performed without pain.

Your operation will be appropriately timed for the arrival of your organ. The anesthesiologist will give you intravenous medication that will put you to sleep. The anesthesia team will monitor your blood pressure, heart rate, breathing, and blood chemistries very closely during the entire operation.

After you are asleep, a breathing tube (endotracheal or ET tube) will be placed in your throat and connected to a machine (ventilator) that will breathe for you while you are asleep. A soft, small tube called a Foley catheter will be inserted into your urinary bladder to drain your urine. A soft tube may also be inserted through your nose or mouth that will go into your stomach; this nasogastric (NG) tube is used to keep your stomach empty to prevent vomiting and choking.

Your surgeon will make an incision that is either shaped like an upside-down "Y" or a hockey stick. The longer portion will be about 12 inches long, extending from the lower right side of the rib cage to just below the breast bone. The shorter portion will be 3 to 4 inches long, extending along the left lower rib cage (Figure 5).

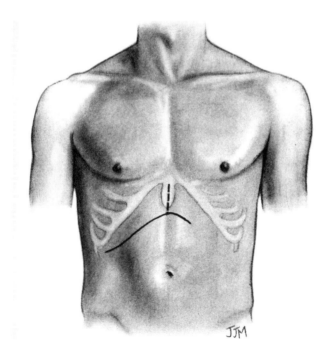

Figure 5   The Upper Abdomen. Illustration courtesy of Roger Jenkins, MD, who holds the rights.

Depending on your liver disease and your physical condition at the time of your transplant, your surgeon will use one of two methods to keep blood away from the liver area (to decrease bleeding) during the operation. In the piggyback technique, the blood vessels around the liver are clamped (held shut) while your new liver is sewn onto a part of your old blood vessel circulation. In a less frequently used procedure called venovenous bypass (Figure 6), a catheter (a small tube) is placed in a vein in your groin. Blood flows through this tube and through a machine that returns the blood to you through a catheter in a vein in your armpit. If the venovenous method is used, you will have two small punctures—in your armpit and in your groin—and a segment of your major blood vessels will be removed along with your old liver.

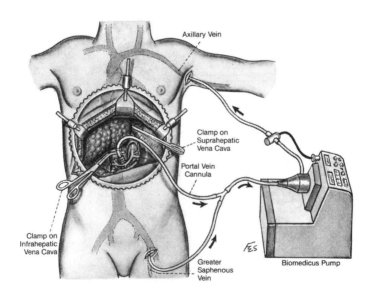

Figure 6   Venovenous Bypass. Image courtesy of Roger Jenkins, MD, who holds the rights.

How your surgeon reconstructs your common bile duct depends on your liver disease. In most instances, the ends of the original common bile duct and the donor common bile duct are sewn together (Figure 7). In this case, a temporary tube or stent is placed in the common bile duct to permit doctors to x-ray the bile ducts after the surgery is complete. This tube is brought outside of your body through a small incision in your abdomen. The part of the tube that remains outside of your body connects to a bag into which the bile—a green/gold-colored fluid produced by your new liver—drains.

Finally, your surgeon will place three drains in your abdomen around your new liver, called Jackson-Pratt drains. One part is inside of your body, and the other is

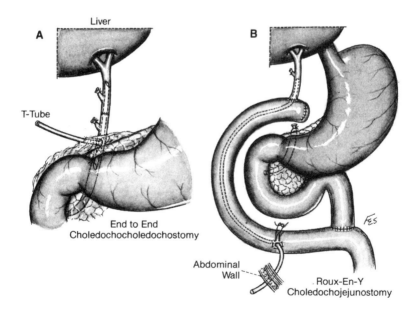

Figure 7 The Bile Ducts after Liver Transplantation. Illustration courtesy of Roger Jenkins, MD, who holds the rights.

outside. The purpose of these drains is to draw excess fluids away from your liver. Your incision will be closed with staples and covered with a gauze dressing. The drains will be attached to your skin to hold them securely in place when you are moved. You will go directly to a post-anesthesia care unit after the operation.

54. How will I feel after I wake up from my transplant surgery?

You will be given general anesthesia for the operation so you will have no recollection of the surgery or the time just prior when you were in the preparation area. After the surgery is complete, you initially go to the post-anes-thesia care unit or to the intensive care unit (ICU) so that the doctors and nurses can monitor you very closely. When you wake up, you may hear unfamiliar sounds, such as the ventilator that may be helping you breathe and the machines that are monitoring your heartbeat, blood pressure, and breathing. You will not be able to talk if you have a breathing tube in place when you awaken. Some medications may make you very sensitive to the noises around you. You might feel nauseated from the anesthesia you were given to put you to sleep; you will be given medication for relief of this nausea. In addition, you may have some pain and discomfort from the surgery and will be given medication to help relieve it. Previous transplant recipients have described the inci-sion pain as very manageable.

The dressing on your incision will be checked fre-quently and may be changed. It is not unusual for flu-ids to drain from your incision for some time after your operation.

Doctors and nurses in the post-anesthesia care unit and ICU will continuously monitor how well your new organ is functioning by taking blood tests, measuring and testing the fluids produced by your body, and using other testing methods, such as x-rays, when necessary and appropriate. When your condition is stable, you will move to the transplant unit for the remainder of your hospital stay.

Remember that many of the tubes, intravenous lines, and monitoring devices that were placed after you went to sleep will still be in place when you wake up. Any drains that were placed during the surgery will be in place as well.

The Breathing Tube (Endotracheal Tube)

The tube that was placed in your throat and attached to the ventilator to help you breathe may still be in place when you wake up. While it is in place, fluid from your mouth and the tube will be removed frequently using a suction device. You will not be able to speak while the ET tube is in place, but your nurse can help you communicate. You may want to establish a way to communicate with your loved ones, such as blinking your eyes once for "yes" and twice for "no." Trying to relax and letting the respirator do the work for you will conserve your energy and make having the tube in place more comfortable. Remember that the ET tube is temporary and necessary for your recovery.

The breathing tube will be removed when the anesthesia has worn off completely and your physicians know that your lungs can function on their own. After a liver transplant, the ET tube usually is removed within 8 to

Endotracheal tube

a tube inserted through the mouth or nose and into the windpipe that enables people to breathe during surgery.

85

24 hours after your surgery. Your doctors and nurses determine when you are ready to breathe on your own by performing a chest x-ray and taking blood samples to measure the oxygen in your blood. After the tube is removed, you may have a mild sore throat; the soreness will disappear in a few days.

After the ET tube is removed, you will be encouraged to cough and breathe deeply very frequently to keep your lungs clear of fluids and to help oxygen flow freely. Having someone support (splint) your stomach and back with a hand or a pillow helps make coughing less painful. Respiratory therapists and your nurses will assist you in keeping your lungs clear with chest therapy (gentle tapping of the lung area) and a spirometer (a device that helps you breathe deeply). All of these precautions are intended to prevent fluid and secretions from collecting in your lungs and causing a lung infection or pneumonia.

The Nasogastric Tube

If an NG tube was inserted through your nose and into your stomach to keep your stomach empty, it still will be in place when you wake up. This tube will be removed when your bowel sounds return or when you pass gas on your own, which usually happens within 24 to 72 hours of your operation.

The Intravenous Lines

The intravenous lines may remain in place for most of your hospital stay. They enable your caregivers to draw your blood for tests, administer any medications that may be needed during your recovery, and provide fluids that help your blood circulate. They also are helpful in monitoring your heart and lung function.

The Foley Catheter

The tube that was placed in your bladder to drain your urine will still be in place when you wake up. It generally is removed a few days after surgery.

The Electrocardiogram Leads

When you leave the post-anesthesia care unit or ICU, the electrocardiogram leads that have been monitoring your heart will be removed.

The Jackson-Pratt Drains

The three Jackson-Pratt drains that your surgeon placed around your new liver will still be in place when you wake up. These tubes enter your abdomen through small incisions. Outside of the body, they look like clear plastic tubes with suction bulbs attached at the end. The fluid in the bulbs may be clear, yellow, or tinged with blood. All of these colors are normal. Generally, two of these drains are removed within 24 hours of your surgery. The remaining Jackson-Pratt drain is removed within 10 days of your surgery.

The Bile Tube

The tube that was placed in your bile ducts will still be in place when you wake up. It permits the doctors to monitor how well your new liver is working and how well the new bile ducts are healing. The bile tube will be clamped shut when a blood test indicates that your bilirubin is less than 3 micromoles per liter as

Bile tube
a tube placed in the bile duct that permits bile to drain into a bag outside of the body.

measured in your blood. It will be removed during an office visit about 8 to 12 weeks after your surgery.

Jonathan's comments:

I remember feeling heavily sedated as I woke up from the transplant. Some close family members were struck by how healthy I looked right after the transplant compared to how compromised I looked before the surgery. This was, of course, due to the healthy lobe of my sister's liver. My immediate recovery was, in fact, somewhat easier than my sister's.

55. How long will I be in the hospital?

The average length of hospitalization after liver transplantation is 10 to 14 days. Some transplant programs are affiliated with "transplant houses" located near the hospital where recipients can recover in a more home-like environment and continue to be followed closely by the transplant team. Placement in a transplant house may allow for an earlier discharge from the hospital.

During the immediate hospitalization after transplantation, you may spend time in the ICU until the ventilator (breathing tube) required during surgery can be removed. Pain medication is administered to control any discomfort from the surgical wound. You will be asked to sit up and even get out of bed with assistance within a day or two after the operation. Food will slowly be re-introduced. Most importantly, immunosuppressive medications will be started and adjusted to prevent rejection of the transplanted liver. When you are able to handle the normal activities of daily living (such as rising from your bed without assistance, showering, and eating), understand your medication regimen, and are medically ready, you will be discharged from the hospital. Sometimes the transplant team and physical therapist may recommend a brief stay in a rehabilitation hospital following the original hospitalization. This can be a very beneficial delay in your return home, because the focus will be on gaining strength and improved nutrition rather than on dealing with medical and surgical issues that often keep you in bed and without food. The improvement in your overall condition in a short time can be dramatic.

56. Are there any early complications I should be aware of?

Your caregivers will be watching for signs of complications so that they may treat them quickly. The most common complications that patients experience are rejection and infection. Other, less common complications are also discussed below.

Rejection

Rejection is a signal that your immune system has identified your new liver as foreign tissue and is trying to get rid of it. Preventing rejection with immunosuppressive medications is the first priority following transplantation. An episode of rejection of the transplanted liver is very common. If rejection occurs, it typically takes place within 5 to 10 days of the transplant operation. The signs you and your doctors and nurses are watching for include a low-grade temperature, decreased appetite, abdominal discomfort, joint and/or back pain, tenderness over the liver, increased abdominal fluid, and feeling like you might have the flu. Other signs include an elevation of your liver function blood tests, a change in the color of your bile (from dark green to light yellow), and a decrease in the amount of bile produced.

Because most people may not have obvious signs of rejection, your liver function tests will be monitored closely. If they are abnormal, a liver **biopsy** may be performed to confirm that you are experiencing a rejection episode. A liver biopsy is accomplished at the hospital bedside. It is rarely painful, although you will feel some pressure when the needle is inserted into the liver (Figure 8). Liver biopsies also can be performed on an outpatient basis. A biopsy may be done if your liver function tests rise after you go home from the hospital.

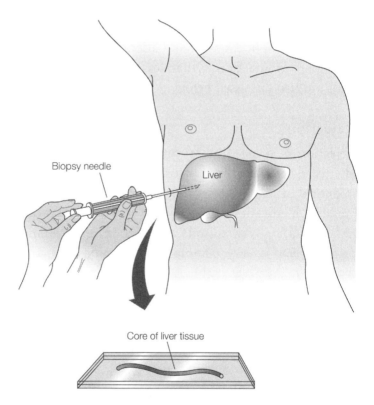

Figure 8   Liver Biopsy

If you have an episode of rejection, the amount of anti-rejection medication will be increased or a different combination of anti-rejection medications will be prescribed. In almost all cases, adjusting the medications will stop the rejection.

Primary Graft Nonfunction

On very rare occasions, a new liver does not function properly or at all after the operation. In such cases, a second transplant operation is necessary.

Infection

The anti-rejection medications that you are taking to prevent and treat rejection tell your immune system to accept your new liver. In doing so, they may also persuade your immune system to accept other foreign invaders that it ordinarily would fight. In other words, the anti-rejection medications can put you at greater risk for developing an infection. The most common infections result from viruses that have been lying dormant in your system or in the donated liver. To prevent infection, you will take antibacterial, antivirus, and antifungal medications for 3 to 6 months after your surgery.

If an infection is suspected, your caregivers may take sputum (the substance coughed up from your lungs), blood, and urine samples, as well as samples from your catheter, wound, and drain sites. Signs of infection may include fever; tiredness or fatigue; diarrhea or vomiting; redness or drainage around your incision, bile, or tube site; or a cough and sore throat. If an infection develops, it will be treated with medication specific for that type of infection. The infectious disease team works with the transplant team to manage and treat infections.

If an infection develops after you have been discharged from the hospital, you may be treated with antibiotics on an outpatient basis. However, some people need to be readmitted for treatment with intravenous medications.

Renal (Kidney) Dysfunction

Sometimes a liver transplant recipient's kidneys do not function as effectively post transplant as they did before the transplant operation. This diminished function could be the result of the long operation, low blood pressure, infection, or the immunosuppressive medications. If your kidneys are not functioning well, they will be monitored closely with blood tests. This complication is usually temporary and reversible.

Bile Duct Complications

The new bile duct that was connected during your surgery may sometimes leak (**bile leak**) or become blocked (**biliary stenosis**) after the operation is complete. The tube that was left in place helps to identify such problems. A painless x-ray called a cholangiogram might be taken to diagnose this complication; it involves injecting contrast dye into the bile tube to identify any leaks or blockages. Most bile duct problems can be treated without further surgery, but some require another operation.

Bile leak

a hole in the bile duct system resulting in bile spilling into the abdomen.

Biliary stenosis

narrowing or constriction of a bile duct.

Stenosis (stricture)

a narrowing of a passage in the body.

Vascular Complications (Problems with Blood Vessels)

On rare occasions, problems may arise with the new connections between the veins and arteries of your new liver and the blood vessels in your body to which they are connected. Laboratory tests and x-rays can help your doctors determine whether such problems are present. Occasionally, surgery is required to repair these problems.

Bleeding

Bleeding from your incision or in your gastrointestinal tract is a potential complication that can be handled easily if identified quickly. Report any bleeding—including bleeding from your incision, throwing up blood, and blood in bowel movements—to your doctor immediately. About 10 percent of people who have liver transplants bleed internally and may need another operation to stop the bleeding.

Thrombosis (Blood Clot)

A blood clot could form in the main artery or vein to the liver. If this happens, the doctors may be able to remove the clot surgically.

57. When will I be able to take care of myself?

Typically, it takes about 3 to 6 months to become fully independent again following a liver transplant. The recipient will not be permitted to drive until all pain medication is stopped and the surgical wounds are healed. The abdominal muscles are necessary to safely operate a car but are cut during surgery. You must allow yourself adequate time to heal and strengthen these muscles before putting pressure on them.

It is important that you have adequate support systems in place following your transplantation procedure. The needs for transportation to and from the transplant center (often on a weekly basis for the first few months after transplantation), preparation of meals, and assistance with administration of medications mean that the recipient will require ongoing help for several months after the surgery.

PART SIX

Recurrent Liver Disease

Can my original disease recur in the new liver?

I was transplanted because of hepatitis C cirrhosis. Will hepatitis C recur in the new liver?

Is there any treatment for hepatitis C after liver transplantation?

More...

58. Can my original disease recur in the new liver?

Liver transplantation was performed because your liver disease caused cirrhosis and later signs of liver failure such as variceal bleeding, ascites, or encephalopathy. In most cases, this process will have taken years to occur. Many liver diseases—particularly inherited diseases such as Wilson's disease and alpha-1 antitrypsin deficiency—are cured by transplantation and therefore do not recur. Other diseases, such as alcoholic liver disease, will not recur as long as the recipient remains sober. Fatty liver disease, also known as non-alcoholic steatohepatitis, may not recur if the recipient maintains adequate weight and blood sugar control after transplantation.

Many of the common liver diseases are due to autoimmune processes. In other words, the immune system identifies the liver cells or bile ducts as foreign tissue and abnormal. It then tries to attack and eliminate the liver. This process results in slow but steady damage to liver and/or bile duct cells and can lead to cirrhosis. Examples of autoimmune liver diseases include autoimmune hepatitis, primary biliary cirrhosis, primary sclerosing cholangitis, and overlap syndrome. The pre-transplant treatment of these conditions is difficult and may involve suppression of the immune system.

After transplantation, there is a risk—estimated to be 5 to 25 percent—that these autoimmune diseases may recur. Of course, there are also several reasons why the disease would *not* recur. After transplantation, the patient takes immunosuppressive drugs, primarily to prevent rejection. Fortunately, these same drugs have a second benefit: They can be effective in controlling autoimmune diseases. A second reason for optimism regarding recurrence relates to the new liver's genetics. Prior to transplantation, the recipient's immune system had recognized its own liver as foreign and developed specific antibodies to attack it. These antibodies may have been capable of recognizing only the native (recipient's own) liver; as a consequence, they may not identify the new liver as foreign. These antibodies are not the same ones that might potentially cause rejection of the transplanted organ.

There are other, equally valid reasons why the autoimmune disease *might* recur in the new liver. First, the antibodies developed for the native liver may, in fact, be able to recognize the new liver as foreign, starting the disease process all over again. Second, the immune system may develop new antibodies to attack the transplanted liver. Third, the transplant team and patient are usually motivated to reduce the immunosuppressive medications in an effort to limit the side effects; as a result, the autoimmune disease may become inadequately controlled by the medications. Lastly, there may be other factors that we are not aware of that cause autoimmune diseases.

59. I was transplanted because of hepatitis C cirrhosis. Will hepatitis C recur in the new liver?

Recurrence of hepatitis C virus (HCV) disease in the transplanted organ occurs in all patients transplanted for HCV-related cirrhosis who still have the virus when they undergo transplantation. This virus is actually detectable in the bloodstream and the new liver as early as during the transplant operation. Typically,

HCV-infected patients will develop elevated liver enzymes and signs of an inflamed liver about 3 to 6 months after the transplant. The majority of these patients have mild to moderate inflammation, minimal to mild scarring of the liver, and acceptable 1- and 5-year survival rates. Most can expect 10 to 20 years of good liver health before significant damage from HCV recurs. A smaller proportion of patients, perhaps 20 to 40 percent, will develop a more rapid progression of HCV liver disease. These patients may develop signs of liver failure 5 to 10 years after the transplant. Even less common (affecting 1 to 5 percent of HCV-infected patients) is fibrosing cholestatic hepatitis, which can destroy the new liver within 1 year. At the present time, we have not identified any pre-transplant features that can predict with certainty which pathway any individual liver transplant recipient with HCV disease will follow.

Patients transplanted with known HCV are monitored in the usual post-transplant fashion. Some transplant programs schedule liver biopsies to occur at predetermined time intervals to get an idea of the rate at which inflammation and scarring are progressing. Other programs biopsy only those patients who develop abnormal liver blood tests. If the biopsy shows significant inflammation or scarring due to recurrent HCV, treatment is considered.

60. Is there any treatment for hepatitis C after liver transplantation?

There are three approaches to treating hepatitis C recurrence after liver transplantation:

Prophylaxis against hepatitis C is the administration of medications to protect the new liver from becoming infected with the virus. Unfortunately, no HCV **antibody** preparations effectively protect the new liver, so this approach is not possible.

The pre-emptive approach calls for treatment of everyone with hepatitis C after transplantation, regardless of the timing or severity of the infection.

Treatment of established recurrent disease is the most commonly applied option.

To date, no study has compared pre-emptive therapy to treatment of established disease. In addition, no data suggest that early treatment during the first clinical signs of recurrent HCV disease influences the natural history of the disease. Based upon the limited available data, the role for pre-emptive antiviral therapy remains to be defined.

A number of recent papers have reported that combination therapy with interferon and ribavirin is associated with a sustained virologic response (cure) rate of 20 to 30 percent in liver recipients with recurrent HCV disease; however, most of these studies were small. One major problem with these studies is the significant variability in the ways that patients were chosen for treatment and immunosuppression, making the interpretation of the results of these studies difficult. Nevertheless, the rate of sustained virologic response seems to be lower than the rate reported for non-transplant HCV patients. In addition, interferon/ribavirin therapy in liver recipients

Prophylaxis

administration of medication that helps prevent disease.

Antibody

a protein molecule produced by the immune system in response to a foreign body, such as virus or a transplanted organ. Because antibodies fight the transplanted organ and try to reject it, recipients are required to take anti-rejection (immunosuppressive) drugs.

Recurrent Liver Disease

with recurrent HCV disease is associated with toxicity of the medications and side effects leading to more frequent dose reductions and discontinuation of therapy.

Many questions remain unanswered with regard to the treatment of post-liver transplant HCV disease, including the timing of treatment, the best treatment regimen, the most effective duration of therapy, and the role of immunosuppression in progressive recurrent HCV disease. Nevertheless, while no firm recommendations can be made, the research conducted to date suggests that a patient with recurrent HCV disease who has stage 2 or higher fibrosis should be given a trial of combination pegylated interferon/ribavirin therapy. Several ongoing studies are currently addressing these issues.

In view of the many unknowns about the natural history of recurrent HCV disease, two approaches to treatment can be suggested. The first approach is to start treatment at the first evidence of acute graft injury (acute recurrent HCV disease), which typically occurs in the first 6 months post transplant. The second approach is to initiate treatment when the patient shows evidence of liver disease based on the results of a liver biopsy. Given that the results of treatment at these two time points, the tolerability of the treatment, and its effectiveness in improving the transplant recipient's health are unknown, it is important to discuss these issues with your transplant team. Your transplant team may already have a preferred approach.

61. I was transplanted because of chronic hepatitis B cirrhosis. Will hepatitis B recur in the new liver?

Although hepatitis B can recur in the new liver, many treatment options are available that can prevent this outcome. In the past, failure to treat recurrent hepatitis B usually resulted in liver failure within 1 year after transplantation. To prevent this outcome, physicians began administering hepatitis B immune globulin (HBIg) to all liver transplant recipients with preexisting hepatitis B. This strategy immediately reduced the recurrence rate from 80 percent to 20 percent. Ongoing administration of this intravenous medication has further reduced the chance of recurrence. Typically, HBIg is given either intravenously or by intramuscular shot once a month indefinitely.

More recently, oral medications to control hepatitis B have become available and are now widely used. These pills are taken once a day and are well tolerated with few, if any, side effects. Currently, standard practice calls for transplant recipients to receive both HBIg and one or two of the oral hepatitis B medications indefinitely so as to prevent recurrence of hepatitis B in the new liver. Studies are looking at whether HBIg is really necessary, with the hope that hepatitis B after liver transplantation may be prevented or controlled with the pills alone.

PART SEVEN

Expectations

What happens after I am discharged
from the hospital?

Can I drink alcohol after my transplant?

How long will my liver last after transplantation?

More...

62. What happens after I am discharged from the hospital?

Even before your surgery took place, the transplant team has made sure you are well prepared to be at home. If you have any questions or concerns, never hesitate to call a transplant team member—the doctor, nurse coordinator, or social worker. You have a lot of information to learn and understand.

After your transplant, you may feel anxious, frightened, and overwhelmed. It will take some time for your energy level to return to normal and for you to settle into the routines you need to follow to stay well. Although other people may assume you are healthy now that the surgery is over, remember that you need to be patient during this recovery phase and follow the advice of your doctors and nurses. You will feel better as time goes on—but it will take time. You may have some setbacks along the way and feel discouraged. Share your feelings with your family, others who are close to you, and your doctors and nurses. If you are concerned about what you are feeling, you may want to consider seeing a mental health professional. If so, your doctors, nurses, or social worker can refer you to someone near your home.

It will take some time for your energy level to return to normal and for you to settle into the routines you need to follow to stay well.

Follow-up Visits

An appointment with a transplant surgeon or physician will be scheduled before you leave the hospital. It is very important to keep this appointment and future appointments so that your progress can be checked, your medications reviewed, and your laboratory tests monitored to confirm that you and your new organ are doing well. You may need blood tests at a laboratory near your home and/or at the hospital between visits as well. Other tests, such as x-rays or a biopsy, may need to be performed at certain times, too. Your visits will typically be scheduled once a week for 1 to 2 months following transplantation. They will then be spaced every 2 weeks, then once a month, then once every 6 to 8 weeks, and finally once every 3 to 6 months. You also may have appointments with your gastroenterologist or primary care physician.

Medicines

You will be taking several medicines following your transplant (described in detail in Part 8). When you leave the hospital, you will be given a medication card that lists which medicines you are taking, what doses to take, and when to take them. At your follow-up visits, your doctor and transplant nurse coordinator will review your medications and discuss any concerns you have, including side effects you might be experiencing. Because medications are sometimes adjusted to achieve the best results with the fewest side effects, it is important to bring your medication card to your follow-up appointments to record any changes.

Your responsibilities regarding your medications are summarized here:

- Make sure that you take your anti-rejection medications, as well as your other medications, at the same time every day.
- If you missed or vomited a dose of your anti-rejection medicine and do not know what to do, call your transplant team.
- Do not use any over-the-counter medicines, except Tylenol (acetaminophen, but no more than 2,000

milligrams in 24 hours), without checking with your doctor or nurse.

- Do not use alcohol, cocaine, heroin, or marijuana—they may put your transplant at risk.
- Call the transplant team if you have any questions or concerns about your medicines.

Your Daily Record

It is wise to keep a daily record of your weight, temperature, frequency of urination and bowel movements, tube drainage, blood sugars (if you are diabetic), and any other notes. You should aim for accuracy when keeping this record, because it will help you identify signs of a problem and will help your doctors and nurses monitor your progress.

Your responsibilities regarding your daily record are summarized here:

- Fill in the information on your daily record sheet consistently and accurately. For example, take your temperature once a day at the same time of day.
- Weigh yourself at the same time every day on the same scale with the same amount of clothing on.
- Check the color and odor of your urine.
- Check your incision and tube site for an increase in redness and unusual drainage. Measure the amount of fluid draining from your tube site if you have one.
- Test your blood sugar at least two times a day: in the morning (this is called a fasting blood sugar) and in the late afternoon (only for those patients who have been advised to do so).
- Be sure to write down all of this information every day.

What to Watch for and When to Call the Transplant Team

While you were in the hospital, your doctors and nurses were constantly watching for signs of a rejection episode, infection, and other problems. Now that you are at home, you need to be a partner in your care and watch for these signs yourself. If you experience any of the following symptoms or if you "just don't feel right," call your transplant team:

- Temperature higher than 100.5 °F
- Flu-like symptoms, such as chills, aches, joint pain, headache, and increased fatigue
- Nausea, vomiting, and diarrhea
- Severe stomach cramps
- Increased pain, redness, or tenderness over your transplant site
- Abnormal drainage near or on your incision
- Very dark or tea-colored urine
- Decrease in the amount of urine or no urine at all
- Pain or burning when urinating
- Frequent urination
- Light or clay-colored stools
- Yellowing of your eyes or skin
- A 6-pound weight gain in less than 3 days
- Abnormal blood sugars (if applicable)
- Sore throat

Here are more reasons to call the transplant team:

- You cannot or did not take your anti-rejection medications.
- Your drainage tube comes out.
- You are short of breath or have chest pain.

Expectations

- You have persistent stomach pain or indigestion.
- You catch a cold or another illness.
- Your urine is cloudy, is bloody, or smells bad.
- You have been exposed to chickenpox, measles, German measles, or mumps and have never had the disease.
- You lose 3 pounds in less than 1 day.
- You have increased swelling in your hands or feet.
- Your doctor changes a medication or prescribes a new medication.
- You have sores or blisters in your mouth.
- You see white spots on your tongue or in your mouth.
- You want to take an over-the-counter medication other than acetaminophen (Tylenol).
- You have questions.

Jonathan's comments:

It was difficult leaving the hospital after the transplant knowing the incredible staff saved my life and now I was venturing home on my own. Even though I had a lot of support, I didn't have the day-to-day medical care. I had so much to learn about my recovery before I could go home. It was scary when I had to rely on so many people to help me with my physical limitations, knowing they couldn't be with me for the long haul. At some point, I had to trust myself and those around me to help me live my life again and celebrate this gift I was given.

63. Can I drink alcohol after my transplant?

Virtually all liver transplant programs prohibit the use of alcohol after transplantation. Much of your own effort and the efforts of your family and physicians will be dedicated to keeping your liver healthy. This program includes proper nutrition, medications, and exercise. The deliberate ingestion of alcohol is in direct opposition to this goal. If your transplanted liver is destroyed by alcohol use, it is extremely unlikely that you would be accepted for a second liver transplant.

64. How long will my liver last after transplantation?

After undergoing liver transplantation, the expectation is that your liver will last for the rest of your life. It has been said that the liver does not age. This explains why it is perfectly acceptable to put a 70-year-old cadaveric donor liver into a 30-year-old recipient. This adage reflects a unique property of the liver: It is the only organ that is capable of regeneration. In other words, damaged liver cells are normally replaced by healthy functional cells. This process does not seem to decrease enough during a lifetime to result in a poorly functioning liver attributable only to the aging process.

Recurrence of liver disease (see Part 6) may limit the liver's ability to function indefinitely in the transplant recipient, however. Other life-limiting factors include conditions common to everyone—for example, heart disease, accidents, stroke, and cancer. To accurately address the question about survival after liver transplantation, several universally accepted milestones have been developed:

- *Operative mortality.* More than 90 percent of patients are still alive 30 days after liver transplanta-

Expectations

tion. The reasons for operative mortality include anesthetic complications, excessive bleeding from varices during the operation, post-operative infections, hepatic artery thrombosis, and primary graft nonfunction (PGNF).

- *One-year mortality.* More than 85 percent of patients are still alive 1 year after transplantation. The typical causes of death during this time frame are infections, delayed hepatic artery thrombosis, and bile duct problems resulting in jaundice and infection.

- *Three-year mortality.* Usually 70 to 80 percent of patients are still alive 3 years after transplantation. Causes of death include recurrent disease, bile duct problems, **chronic rejection**, and, less likely, infections.

- *Five-year mortality.* Approximately 60 to 70 patients are still alive 5 years after transplantation. Recurrent disease, chronic rejection, heart disease, and kidney failure are the major causes of death in this group.

- *Ten-year mortality.* Approximately 45 to 60 percent of patients are still alive 10 years after transplantation. Recurrent disease, chronic rejection, accidents, heart disease, stroke, kidney problems, and other cancers are the primary causes of death.

Note that after 10 years, approximately 50 percent of liver transplant recipients are still alive. To have assessed this group for survival, by definition they must have been transplanted in the early to mid-1990s. Since that time, we have seen many advances in surgical techniques, post-operative care, intensive care unit care, and immunosuppression. Additionally, transplant physicians have become more aware of long-term complications and, therefore, manage these problems more aggressively

Chronic rejection

slow, continuous immunological attack by the host immune system on the transplanted organ, usually resulting in progressive loss of organ function.

than in the past. It is expected that liver transplant recipients from the 2000s will have better long-term survival than their counterparts from the 1990s.

65. Can I go back to my usual routine, like work and exercise, after transplantation?

You will need time to regain your strength and endurance after your transplant, but eventually your activity level should get back to normal. It may take anywhere from 6 weeks to 6 months before you regain enough strength to return to work or to school. It might be possible to reduce your hours when you first return to work. Follow these guidelines when you get home:

- Do the muscle-toning exercises that you began in the hospital two times every day.
- Do not lift anything that weighs more than 10 to 15 pounds—including babies, children, and groceries—until you have been home from the hospital for 2 months. After 2 months, you may gradually begin to lift heavier items if it does not cause discomfort around your incision.
- Walking and stair climbing are excellent exercises for maintaining muscle tone and strength. Consider walking 5 to 10 minutes a day when you first get home, slowly increasing the time you walk each week.
- Do not engage in any strenuous exercise, such as contact sports, jogging, tennis, or body conditioning (weightlifting, push-ups, sit-ups) for at least 2 months

You will need time to regain your strength and endurance after your transplant, but eventually your activity level should get back to normal.

111

after you go home. Talk to your transplant doctor or nurse before you resume these types of activities.

- It is normal to tire easily. Pace yourself and rest when you are tired.
- Talk to your transplant team before you make any travel plans. They can help you maintain the routines you need to follow when you are away and instruct you on what to do if you need medical attention. They also can give you guidelines that will help you avoid infection and other problems when you are away from home.

You can resume sexual activity as soon as you feel able; there are no restrictions. Because you have been through a difficult surgery and are still recovering, it may take several months for your level of sexual desire to return to what you and your partner consider acceptable. Some medicines you are taking might also interfere with sexual functioning. Talk to your transplant team or primary care physician about any problems or concerns you may have. If you are sexually active and do not have a regular partner, you should practice safe sex by using condoms to reduce your risk of sexually transmitted diseases, such as chlamydia, syphilis, **herpes**, hepatitis, gonorrhea, and acquired immune deficiency virus.

Herpes

a family of viruses that can infect humans and can cause lip sores, genital sores, and shingles.

66. Can I get another transplant if I need it?

Depending on the reason you need a second (or third) transplant, you might be a candidate for retransplantation. One reason for early retransplantation is PGNF. PGNF occurs when an acceptable donor liver is transplanted into a recipient but the liver does not perform adequately. In such a case, the patient usually develops liver failure within 7 days of the transplant. PGNF is a very rare occurrence (less than 2 percent of transplants) and has no known cause. In this circumstance the recipient can be placed on the transplant waiting list as Status 1.

A second early cause of retransplantation is hepatic artery thrombosis. In rare cases, during or immediately after the transplant operation the hepatic artery (one of the two blood sources for the liver) may become blocked by a blood clot. The result may be rapid deterioration in liver function, often necessitating retransplantation. If this hepatic artery thrombosis is identified within the first two weeks of transplantation, the patient may be placed on the waiting list as Status 1.

Later causes of retransplantation include chronic rejection, infection with cytomegalovirus, recurrent hepatitis C, bile duct damage, and other recurrent diseases. The decision to retransplant in these settings is difficult, because the results of retransplantation are far inferior to the outcomes with original transplants. The initial surgery will have created adhesions (bands of scar tissue) around the new liver, making it difficult to remove. Also, the effects of progressive liver disease while on immunosuppressive medications seem to be more severe than the liver disease alone. Under the Model of End-Stage Liver Disease (MELD) scoring system, patients with liver failure that occurs *after* transplantation are far sicker than the patients with similar MELD scores who have not yet been transplanted. The 1-year survival rate after initial liver transplantation exceeds 85 percent, whereas the 1-year survival rate for retransplant recipients is only 50 percent.

Expectations

The decision to retransplant patients with recurrent HCV is controversial. Many reports suggest that the 1-year survival rate in this group is only 10 to 40 percent. The rapidity with which hepatitis C destroys the new liver may play a role in the outcome (that is, redeveloping cirrhosis from HCV after 3 years is worse than disease that recurs after 10 years). Many transplant programs have developed policies regarding retransplantation for recurrent HCV; these policies often take into account a variety of factors, including the time since the first transplant, the overall degree of patient illness, the degree of kidney function, and the regional supply of livers.

67. Do I need to avoid anything after liver transplantation?

The following are things you can do (or avoid doing) that will decrease your chance of an infection developing. Your transplant doctor or nurse will tell you when some of these restrictions may be lifted.

- Stay away from people who are obviously sick with the flu or a cold.
- Wash your hands with soap and water before you eat and after you go to the bathroom.
- Shower or bathe regularly. Wash your incision as you would any other part of your body. Do not use lotions or powders on your incision.
- Clean cuts and scrapes with soap and water, and apply an antiseptic and a bandage to them.
- Do not, under any circumstances, change the litter in the cat box or bird cage without gloves. This could cause a serious infection.
- Do not garden, dig in dirt, or mow the lawn without gloves for 6 to 8 weeks after your transplant. This could cause a serious infection.

- Brush and floss your teeth daily.
- Keep your fingernails and toenails clean and trimmed. If your toenails are hard to manage or are ingrown, see a foot specialist.
- Talk to your doctor about getting the flu vaccine and the pneumonia vaccine. These do not contain a live virus and are safe for you to receive.
- Do not get any vaccine that contains a live virus, such as the smallpox or polio vaccine.
- Talk to your doctor if someone in your house will receive a live virus, such as the oral polio vaccine or diphtheria vaccine, if you have not already been vaccinated.
- Do not expose yourself to smoke—either first hand or second hand.
- Do not use alcohol.

68. Which doctors will take care of me after my transplant?

Your liver transplant team will monitor you for the rest of your life but will soon become a *part* of your health-care team rather than *all* of it. Each transplant program follows its patients indefinitely as required by the United Organization for Organ Sharing, but the follow-up schedule may vary by program, distance to the program, your health, and the time since transplantation.

At some point within the first year after transplantation, your transplant-related issues will stabilize: You will experience fewer medication changes, a decreased risk of rejection and post-operative complications, and improved overall health. At this point you will return to the care of your primary care physician to continue your routine health maintenance such as blood pressure monitoring and physical examinations. For regular checkups and common medical problems, such as a cold or the flu, you will see your primary care doctor. He or she needs to be aware that you have undergone a transplant so that when symptoms arise, he or she can determine whether those symptoms are signs of problems related to your transplant or something else. Your primary care physician also needs to be sure that any medications prescribed for you will not interfere with the medications you take to prevent rejection of your new liver.

Because patients on immunosuppressive medications have an increased risk of developing skin cancers, you should see a dermatologist every year for a full body skin examination. This step is important even if you never had a skin cancer before transplantation.

Good dental hygiene is very important after your transplant. Brush your teeth after each meal and at bedtime. Floss your teeth gently every day. *Do not plan any routine dental work until 6 months after your transplant operation.* Visit your dentist every 6 months. Make sure the dentist knows which anti-rejection medications you are taking before he or she does any dental work. You will need to take an antibiotic before having dental work to avoid developing a serious infection. Your dentist knows the guidelines for antibiotic use before dental work. Amoxicillin is the drug of choice. People who are allergic to penicillins can take clindamycin (Cleocin) instead of amoxicillin. People who are taking cyclosporine, tacrolimus, or sirolimus should not take erythromycin, azithromycin (Zithromax), clarithromycin (Biaxin), or dirithromycin (Dynabac). Cyclosporine (Sandimmune, Neoral, Gengraf, Eon) can cause an overgrowth of your gum tissue, which can become swollen and painful. Ask your dentist to suggest oral hygiene measures to relieve the discomfort.

Special Health Issues for Women

The following information is specific to questions and concerns of women:

- Have a Papanicolaou smear once a year.
- Perform a breast self-examination (BSE) every month. The best time to perform a BSE is 1 week after your period ends.
- If you are sexually active and likely to become pregnant, use contraception each time you have intercourse after your transplant. The diaphragm, with a spermicidal gel, or a condom (used correctly) is recommended. Oral birth control pills are not recommended immediately after transplant but may be approved by your doctor at a later time. Be sure to discuss your method of birth control with your transplant doctor or nurse.
- Women may produce eggs 2 to 6 months after the transplant operation but before their regular menstrual periods begin. (This is why birth control is recommended.)
- Women are encouraged to avoid pregnancy for at least 1 year after a transplant operation and at any time if taking mycophenolate mofetil (CellCept, Myfortic). If you discover that you are pregnant at any time after your transplant, contact your transplant team. It is possible to have a normal pregnancy after a transplant, but it should be carefully planned.

- If you use tampons, choose the smallest size needed to meet your needs. Change tampons frequently to avoid infection. Do not use a tampon overnight.
- Women over the age of 50 years should discuss having a screening colonoscopy with a doctor.

Special Health Issues for Men

The following information is specific to the questions and concerns of men:

- Men should perform a self-examination of the testes every month. Call your doctor if you see or feel any abnormal or unusual lumps.
- Men who are age 40 years or older should have a physical examination every year. During the physical examination, you should be screened for prostate cancer.
- Although men may father children at any time, talk to your doctor before trying to conceive to be sure the medicines you are taking, such as mycophenolate mofetil (CellCept, Myfortic), will not affect the baby.
- Men over the age of 50 years should discuss having a screening colonoscopy with a doctor.

69. Will I have to change my diet after transplantation?

A healthy diet plays a significant role by enhancing your ability to heal after surgery.

A healthy diet plays a significant role by enhancing your ability to heal after surgery. This is true not only for transplant recipients but for anyone undergoing surgery. After transplantation, it is important to control your weight and watch your cholesterol—just like other people without medical problems. After you receive your new liver, you will probably be on far fewer dietary restrictions that you had before transplantation. The transplant dietitian will help you design a diet that encourages healthy choices.

You will probably find that you have a better appetite after transplantation than you did before the surgery. In fact, weight gain following transplantation is very common. Some of this weight gain is attributable to the immunosuppressive medications—in particular, prednisone. Fortunately, many transplant programs taper prednisone off very quickly after the operation, so the weight impact of this medication should be short-lived. Maintaining a normal weight will help you avoid other problems common to obesity, such as diabetes, heart disease, and **hypertension**.

Hypertension
high blood pressure. It can cause damage to the body by over-working the heart and blood vessels.

Proteins are critical in wound healing and muscle building, so you must ensure that you eat enough protein to support these functions. Typically, this means 1.2 to 1.4 grams of protein for every 1 kilogram (2.2 pounds) of body weight every day. Proteins are found in meats, poultry, fish, eggs, nuts, and beans. Some patients may have been advised to decrease their protein intake prior to transplantation because of difficulty with hepatic encephalopathy. If this was the case, the protein restriction can be lifted immediately after transplantation.

Carbohydrates are necessary for fuel and energy. Prednisone alters the body's metabolism of carbohydrates, which accounts for much of the weight gain observed after transplantation. Eating fewer "simple" carbohydrates like sugars and sweets will decrease the tendency toward weight gain. "Complex" carbohydrates like cereals, vegetables, whole-grain pasta, bread, rice, and potatoes are healthier choices.

You can eat fats after transplantation, but should restrict your consumption, because fats may adversely affect your cholesterol levels and weight. Saturated fats will have the most negative impact. Sticking to skim milk, low-fat dairy products, and vegetable oils (rather than lard) will help you maintain your weight and keep your cholesterol levels under control. Some immuno-suppressive medications (such as cyclosporine and sirolimus) will increase your cholesterol levels. Because these are necessary medications following transplanta-tion, it is important that you control your cholesterol levels by other means (diet and possibly medication).

Sodium (salt) is found in many foods, but particularly processed foods. Prior to transplantation, you may have been placed on a restricted-sodium diet to limit your fluid retention. After transplantation, fluid reten-tion will not be as much of a problem, but you should still limit your sodium intake to some degree. Fluid retention causes hypertension, another problem com-monly associated with immunosuppressive drugs (for example, cyclosporine and tacrolimus).

70. When can I resume driving after the operation?

Some medicines you are taking can have side effects that affect your ability to drive safely. Therefore, you should not drive immediately after leaving the hospi-tal. You and your doctors must be sure that these side effects—which may include tremors, muscle weakness, and blurry vision—are under control before you take the wheel. You also must be sure your attention is focused on the road and not on your incision. Any pain medication you are taking may interfere with your concentration or ability to stay awake while driving. Be sure to check with your transplant team before you start to drive again. This is an issue of safety for you and others on the road.

71. Will my fatigue get any better after the transplant?

Fatigue is extremely common among patients with liver disease and cirrhosis. It is difficult to gauge the degree of fatigue because each person has different abilities, stamina, and expectations of his or her body. A multitude of factors contribute to a person's overall energy level or, conversely, fatigue level. Elements that improve energy include proper nutrition, moderate exercise, good sleep habits, minimal stress, and appropriate use of medications. Factors that increase fatigue include chronic liver disease itself, certain medications such as narcotics and diuretics, poor nutrition, excess weight, inability to exercise, depression, and poor sleep. Of course, many of these factors are associated with cirrhosis and liver failure, so it is not surprising that fatigue is a prominent symptom of these conditions.

After transplantation, you may continue to experience fatigue for quite some time, but your energy level should gradually improve. There are new reasons for diminished energy after transplant surgery. First, it takes time for the surgical wounds to heal. During the operation, the surgeons will cut the vertical abdominal muscles in two. These muscles are necessary to perform a sit-up and are essential for holding the body upright when walking, shifting in bed, and rising from a seated position. It takes about 6 months for these muscles to return to their normal strength. In the meantime, your body will use different muscles to perform these tasks, but this shift requires additional energy expenditure. In addition, many of the medications prescribed after transplantation can cause fatigue as a side effect. Some of these medications will be stopped, such as pain medications, or decreased over time, such as prednisone.

Your expectations after transplantation also play a role in your perception of fatigue. Years of liver disease and cirrhosis may have taken a physical toll on your body prior to your latest surgery. Although transplantation should stop the progression of this decline, it will not immediately restore you to your health of many years earlier, nor will it reverse the aging process. It is best to have reasonable expectations and set feasible goals with regard to return of energy. To this end, focus on those elements you can control. Proper nutrition, exercise, and sleep are critical. Work closely with your transplant team to address any medication concerns and reduce those medications that contribute to fatigue. Lastly, minimize your level of stress if possible.

72. I was asked to participate in a research study. Is this a good idea?

Research is an important component of most liver transplant programs. New surgical techniques, medications, immunosuppressive regimens, and post-transplant treatments for viral hepatitis require rigorous testing before they can be accepted as the standard of care. Because of the diversity of the patients affected by liver disease and the relatively few liver transplants performed in the United States each year, many of the questions that might advance the care of liver transplant recipients remain unanswered.

Participation in research requires **informed consent**. The informed consent process offers many benefits for the patient. Good researchers will explain their research and the process so that you understand it and do not feel like a "guinea pig." Informed consent implies that the patient understands the research proposal and the rationale for it (that is, the question that the researcher is trying to answer). It details the research protocol, its risks, and its potential benefits. In addition, the patient must understand the alternatives to research and the current standard of care. Once the patient has demonstrated an understanding of these issues, he or she may choose to participate in research by giving true informed consent. If the individual has any reluctance to participate or the research does not proceed as expected, consent can be withdrawn at any time without penalty. The patient can then discuss the alternatives with his or her doctor or return to the accepted standard of medical care.

Informed consent
a person's voluntary agreement, based on adequate knowledge and understanding of relevant information, to participate in research or to undergo a diagnostic, therapeutic, or preventive procedure.

73. Can I meet the family of my liver donor?

Recipients of donated organs often want to find out specifics about the person who donated the organ they received. In contrast, one of the basic tenets of organ donation is anonymity. This secrecy is necessary to protect the surviving family members' privacy. The donor family has likely experienced a traumatic event and the premature loss of a loved one. They may not be ready to meet a stranger who is living because of their loss. Sometimes, at a later date, many families who donate their relative's organs wish to know where and to whom the organs went.

Although there are no laws that prohibit donors and recipients from meeting, all organ procurement organizations (OPOs) have established privacy policies to protect both parties to the donation. However, this right to privacy may be waived if the two groups agree to meet.

The mechanism for meeting is initiated by writing a letter. The recipient is encouraged to write a letter to the donor family expressing his or her gratitude, hopes, and wishes for the future. The OPO, during its post-donation discussion with the donor family, makes them aware that the recipient may write letters to the donor family that will be kept at the OPO. Some families leave instructions with the OPO to not forward any such letters, because they do not want to re-experience the pain of losing their loved one. If the donor family wishes to know whether a letter is waiting for them, they can contact the OPO. The OPO will then forward the letter with all names removed. If the two parties interact frequently (always via the OPO), they may choose to meet. In these special circumstances where both parties want to meet and talk, and both waive the right to privacy, a joint session is occasionally arranged by the OPO with the assistance of a specially trained chaperone.

A meeting between the donor family and the recipient can have long-lasting, powerful effects on both. Sometimes, bonds are made and communication is frequent. At other times, the interaction is uncomfortable and terminated. Remember—every family grieves differently.

74. Can I father a child or give birth after a liver transplant?

The goal of liver transplantation is to return patients with liver disease to a normal life. This includes the ability to conceive a child. Many transplant recipients have children after transplant surgery. Female transplant recipients should wait at least 1 year after a transplant before becoming pregnant. Male transplant recipients should wait until they are fully recovered from surgery before fathering a child. Because there are increased risks for mothers (rejection and transplant organ loss) and babies (premature births and low birthweight), preconception counseling with an obstetrician who specializes in high-risk pregnancies and with the transplant team is recommended. Some anti-rejection medications, especially mycophenolate mofetil (Cell-Cept) and mycophenolate sodium (Myfortic), are potentially harmful to a fetus.

Let the transplant team know if you are planning to become a parent to see whether your medications can be changed before conception. The decision to become a parent should be made only after you fully appreciate the risks involved.

Expectations

PART EIGHT

Medications

Why are immunosuppressive drugs necessary?

What are the immunosuppressive drugs?

Will I ever be able to stop my
immunosuppressive drugs?

More...

75. Why are immunosuppressive drugs necessary?

Anti-rejection medications (immunosuppressants) are prescribed to help your immune system accept your new organ. Your transplant team may prescribe any of several anti-rejection medications: cyclosporine, tacrolimus, prednisone, mycophenolate, azathioprine, sirolimus, OKT3, and basiliximab or daclizumab. Some are taken in pill form every day; others are administered intravenously. As long as you have a functioning transplanted organ, you will take one or more anti-rejection medications for the rest of your life. Following the dosing schedule determined by your transplant team is essential to your well-being. Your transplant team will determine the appropriate medications for you. You may be asked to participate in a self-medication program while you are in the hospital. By taking responsibility for your own medications in the hospital while under the supervision of a nurse, you can make the transition to home less stressful. Remember, *taking your medications is your responsibility*.

As long as you have a functioning transplanted organ, you will take one or more anti-rejection medications for the rest of your life.

Jonathan's comments:

When I take my anti-rejection medication, it is troubling to know there are many side effects. The risks of not being responsible with this medication far outweigh the side effects. I feel it is my responsibility to the transplant team, my family, my sister who donated, and me to take precious care of the "gift of life" that has allowed me to live out my life.

76. What are the immunosuppressive drugs?

Immunosuppressive drugs decrease the function of your immune system so that your immune system does not react to (that is, reject) the new liver. Without immuno-suppressive drugs, the immune system would recognize the new organ as foreign and attack it.

The following list includes the commonly prescribed immunosuppressive agents and their side effects. After transplantation you will be prescribed several, but not all, of these medications.

Cyclosporine

Cyclosporine (also called Neoral, Sandimmune, Gen-graf, Eon) is a primary immunosuppressive agent that is classified as a calcineurin inhibitor. This drug has been in use to prevent rejection in transplant recipients for more than 30 years.

Notes about Cyclosporine

- You should not stop taking cyclosporine or change the dose or the time at which you take it unless your transplant team instructs you to do so.
- Cyclosporine should be taken in the morning and at night, about 12 hours apart. Some patients need only one dose daily.
- The amount of cyclosporine in your blood will be monitored by blood tests. Do not take cyclosporine on the day you are having blood tests until after the blood is drawn.
- Always take the correct dose of cyclosporine after your blood has been drawn.
- Cyclosporine may interact with some commonly used medications, such as antibiotics and high blood pressure medications. It is very important that you check with the transplant team before starting any new medications, especially antibiotics.

Possible Side Effects

Hand tremors or shaking; numbness or tingling in the hands, feet, mouth, or lips; decreased ability of the body to fight infection; abnormal kidney function tests; high blood pressure; swollen gums; hair growth; runny nose; high cholesterol; upset stomach; headache; increased risk of certain types of cancer, such as skin cancer, cervical cancer, and rarely lymphoma (lymph node cancer)

Tacrolimus

Tacrolimus (Prograf, FK-506) is also a primary immunosuppressive agent and, like cyclosporine, a calcineurin inhibitor. It is newer than cyclosporine and was approved for use in the United States in 1995. Tacrolimus is never used in conjunction with cyclosporine.

Notes about Tacrolimus

- You should not stop taking tacrolimus or change the dose or the time at which you take it unless your transplant team instructs you to do so.
- Tacrolimus should be taken in the morning and at night, about 12 hours apart.
- The amount of tacrolimus in your blood will be monitored by blood tests. Do not take tacrolimus on the day you are having blood tests done until after the blood is drawn.
- Always take the correct dose of tacrolimus after your blood has been drawn.
- Tacrolimus may interact with some commonly used medications, such as antibiotics and high blood pressure medications. It is important that you check with the transplant team before starting any new medications.

Possible Side Effects

Headaches; nausea; diarrhea; stomach cramps; hand tremors or shaking; high blood sugar; high blood **potassium**; abnormal kidney function; hair loss; sleep disturbances; numbness and tingling in hands, feet, and mouth; decreased ability of the body to fight infection; increased risk of certain types of cancer, such as skin cancer, cervical cancer, and rarely lymphoma (lymph node cancer)

Potassium

an electrolyte responsible for vital muscle functions.

Prednisone

Prednisone (Deltasone, Orasone) is an immunosuppressant and anti-inflammatory medication. Although this drug is associated with many side effects, it remains an essential part of most post-transplant immunosuppressive regimens. You will receive your first dose of prednisone intravenously during the transplant operation.

Notes about Prednisone

- Do not stop taking prednisone or change the dose or the time at which you take it unless your transplant team instructs you to do so. A sudden discontinuation of prednisone can result in a severe illness called adrenal insufficiency.
- Always take prednisone with food or milk.
- If you have an episode of rejection, you may be instructed to take higher doses of prednisone.

Possible Side Effects

Increased appetite; acne; bruising; muscle weakness (especially in the upper legs and arms); stomach irritation; increased body and facial hair; mood change; decreased ability of the body to fight infections; high blood sugar; visual changes; delayed wound healing;

softening of bones (osteoporosis); fluid and salt retention; anxiety; cataracts; glaucoma; night sweats;
increased risk of certain cancers; menstrual irregularity

Mycophenolate

Mycophenolate mofetil (CellCept) and mycophenolate sodium (Myfortic) belong to a class of medications called antiproliferative drugs. These drugs are
typically used in addition to a primary agent such as a
calcineurin inhibitor.

Notes about Mycophenolate

- Do not stop taking mycophenolate or change the
  dose or the time at which you take it unless your
  transplant team instructs you to do so.
- Always swallow the capsules whole. Do not crush
  them, chew them, or open them.
- If a capsule comes apart, do not inhale the powder and do not let the powder touch your skin. If
  the powder touches your skin, wash your skin
  thoroughly with soap and water. If the powder
  comes in contact with your eyes, rinse them well
  with water.
- Do not take mycophenolate with **antacids** that
  contain magnesium or aluminum, such as
  Mylanta.
- Stomach cramps, nausea, and diarrhea may be
  controlled by spreading the dosage of mycophenolate mofetil over the course of the day. Ask
  your transplant team if this is an option for you.
  Do not make any changes in your medication
  schedule before talking with them.

Antacid

a medicine that pro-
tects the digestive
system. It can relieve
indigestion and other
digestive discomfort.

- You will have regular blood tests to monitor the effects of mycophenolate on your white blood cell count.
- Take mycophenolate 2 hours after cyclosporine or tacrolimus.
- Do not become pregnant or father a child while taking mycophenolate.

Possible Side Effects

Nausea; vomiting; diarrhea; stomach cramps; gas; decrease in appetite; decreased ability of the body to fight infection; increased risk of certain types of cancers, such as skin cancer, cervical cancer, and lymphoma (lymph node cancer)

Azathioprine

Azathioprine (Imuran) is an antiproliferative agent that is similar to mycophenolate mofetil. The two drugs are never used together.

Notes about Azathioprine

- Do not stop taking azathioprine or change the dose or the time at which you take it unless your transplant team instructs you to do so.
- You will have regular blood tests to monitor the effects of azathioprine on your white blood cell count.
- Do not take allopurinol (Zyloprim) for gout while taking azathioprine without discussing this issue with the transplant team.
- Women should avoid pregnancy while taking azathioprine. Contact your transplant team if you do become pregnant.

Possible Side Effects

Decreased ability of the body to fight infection; abnormal liver function tests (very rare); mouth sores; thinning hair; nausea; vomiting; bruising; increased risk of certain cancers, such as skin cancer, cervical cancer, and lymphoma (lymph node cancer)

Sirolumus

Sirolumus (Rapamune, Rapamycin) is another immunosuppressant that is similar in chemical structure to tacrolimus. It does not cause kidney dysfunction but cannot be used immediately after liver transplantation because it delays healing of the surgical wound and rarely causes blood clots in the artery leading to the liver. Sirolumus is sometimes used several months or years after transplantation in patients who are at risk of kidney failure. It can be used in combination with low doses of cyclosporine or tacrolimus.

Notes about Sirolumus

- Take sirolumus 4 hours after cyclosporine or tacrolimus.
- Sirolimus comes in liquid and pill form. The liquid can be mixed only with water or orange juice and must be placed in a glass or plastic container.
- Sirolumus comes in a multidose bottle or single-dose foil pouches.
- Sirolumus liquid should be kept refrigerated.

Possible Side Effects

Triglycerides

a form of fat that the body makes from sugar, alcohol, and excess calories.

Elevated cholesterol and **triglycerides**; high blood pressure; rash; acne; anemia; joint pain; low potassium; low white blood cells; low platelets; anemia; diarrhea

Muromonab-CD3

Muromonab (OKT3) is a rarely used immunosuppressant. Its primary use is to treat acute rejection that has not responded to standard treatment with prednisone.

Notes about Muromonab

- Orthoclone OKT3 can be given only intravenously (through a vein). This drug does not come in pill form. It usually is given at the hospital once a day for 5 to 14 days.
- If you receive Orthoclone OKT3, the purpose is to prevent or to treat a rejection episode.
- Tylenol and/or Benadryl will be given before the OKT3 to help prevent some of the side effects.

Possible Side Effects

Decreased ability of the body to fight infection; fever; nausea; vomiting; diarrhea; shortness of breath; increased risk of certain types of cancer, such as skin cancer, cervical cancer, and lymphoma (lymph node cancer)

Basiliximab

Basiliximab (Simulect) is a monoclonal antibody directed against parts of the immune system that cause acute rejection.

Notes about Basiliximab

- Basiliximab is used to prevent (but not to treat) episodes of acute rejection.
- Basiliximab can only be given intravenously.
- The first dose is usually administered in the operating room during the transplant operation.
- A second dose of basiliximab is typically given intravenously 4 days after the operation.

Possible Side Effects

Acne; constipation; nausea; diarrhea; headache; heartburn; trouble sleeping; weight gain; excessive hair growth; muscle or joint pain

Daclizumab

Daclizumab (Zenapax) is a monoclonal antibody directed against parts of the immune system that cause acute rejection.

Notes about Daclizumab

- Daclizumab is used to prevent (but not to treat) episodes of acute rejection.
- Daclizumab can only be given intravenously.
- The first dose is usually administered in the operating room during the transplant operation.
- A second dose of daclizumab is typically given intravenously 4 days after the operation.

Possible Side Effects

Chest pain; coughing; dizziness; fever; nausea; rapid heart rate; shortness of breath; swelling of the feet or lower legs; trembling or shaking of the hands or feet; vomiting; weakness

77. Will I ever be abe to stop my immunosuppressive drugs?

Much of the success of liver transplantation can be attributed to improvements in the immunosuppressive drugs prescribed after the surgery. When the only drugs available were prednisone and azathioprine, the rejection rates and risk of graft loss were very high. Long-term survival was unusual. With the introduction of cyclosporine, however, patient survival increased almost immediately. The availability of even more drugs has since expanded the choices for safe and effective immunosuppression. Unfortunately, current immunosuppressive medications have a number of undesirable side effects (see Question 76).

Now that rejection has become a rare and controllable phenomenon, researchers are trying to determine the lowest amount of immunosuppression that will prevent rejection and graft loss while at the same time minimizing the drugs' side effects. The advent of powerful primary agents, such as tacrolimus and sirolimus, has allowed us to decrease the overall number of drugs needed in one individual for adequate immunosuppression. The agent most commonly targeted for reduction has been prednisone—the drug with the most frequent and problematic side effects. The reduction in the use of prednisone has decreased the frequency of elevated blood sugars, osteoporosis, weight gain, and edema following transplantation. Many patients with no prior episodes of acute or chronic rejection, adequate kidney function, and acceptable liver function tests are able to stop taking prednisone altogether. With the addition of mycophenolate to the primary agent, even patients with a history of mild rejection and kidney dysfunction may be candidates to stop prednisone therapy.

A small number of reports from transplant centers have indicated that all immunosuppressive drugs may be stopped in a select group of transplant recipients.

These reports emphasize the "success stories" and de-emphasize the failures and their outcomes—rejection, graft loss, retransplantation, or death. The difficulty arises in choosing the appropriate patient for total drug withdrawal. At this time, we do not have any blood tests or markers that can reliably identify the best patients for removal of immunosuppression. Because the risks are so high (for example, graft loss), most transplant programs will not entertain the possibility of total immunosuppression withdrawal.

78. I thought I'd be able to stop many of the medications I took before the transplant. Why am I still taking so many medications?

You may be able to stop many of the medications you were taking before your transplant. Because of the multitude of risks and side effects caused by the immunosuppressive drugs, however, you will need to take additional medications to minimize their risks and control the side effects. The immunosuppressive drugs decrease the function of your immune system. As a result, common viruses and bacteria, which are typically kept at bay by the intact immune system, may now cause serious infections. These potential infections include cytomegalovirus (**CMV**) and *Pneumocystis carinii* pneumonia (**PCP**).

CMV is a common virus that is similar to infectious mononucleosis. It may cause no symptoms or perhaps a febrile illness. When the immune system is intact, you can get CMV only once. However, in the immunosuppressed patient, the virus can re-emerge

CMV (cytomegalovirus)

a virus that lies dormant in the body and can be reactivated after transplantation, causing a flu-like illness, pneumonia, and/or gastrointestinal ulcers.

PCP (Pneumocystis carinii pneumonia)

a type of pneumonia that is most often seen in patients whose immune systems are suppressed (as by immunosuppressive medications).

and cause inflammation in the new liver, kidney problems, pneumonia, and blood problems. *Pneumocystis carinii* infection usually causes pneumonia if it occurs in transplant recipients. Because these infections can be devastating or even fatal after transplantation, medications are prescribed to significantly reduce the risk of occurrence. As time goes by after transplantation, many of these preventive medications can be stopped as the degree of immunosuppression required to prevent rejection decreases.

Anti-infection Medications (Antibacterials)

Antibacterials (also called antibiotics) are prescribed to prevent and treat bacterial infections. Because anti-rejection medications can weaken your immune system, you are at more risk for the development of an infection, especially in your urinary tract or lungs. Antibiotics may be prescribed to decrease your chances of an infection developing and definitely will be prescribed if an infection develops. Several antibiotics are commonly prescribed, including trimethoprim-sulfamethoxazole, levofloxacin, and ciprofloxacin.

Trimethoprim-sulfamethoxazole (TMP-SMZ, Bactrim, Cotrim, Septra) is prescribed to prevent PCP. It is usually continued for 3 months after transplantation.

Notes about Trimethoprim-Sulfamethoxazole

- TMP-SMZ is available as a pill or a liquid.
- Take TMP-SMZ with 8 ounces of water.
- Do not take TMP-SMZ if you are allergic to sulfa.

- TMP-SMZ may be used to treat a **urinary tract infection** or pneumonia.
- Tell your transplant team if you become pregnant while taking TMP-SMZ.

Possible Side Effects

Low white blood cell count, nausea, vomiting, rash, itching, loss of appetite, abnormal kidney function tests

Levofloxacin (Levaquin) and **ciprofloxacin** (Cipro) are antibiotics with many uses. They are effective therapy for some types of pneumonia (but not PCP), urinary tract infections, and bacterial cholangitis (infection of the bile ducts). Levofloxacin and ciprofloxacin are typically not used as preventive medicine but rather as a treatment.

Notes about Levofloxacin and Ciprofloxacin

- Drink a lot of fluids when taking levofloxacin or ciprofloxacin.
- Tell your transplant team if you have hives, a skin rash, or ringing in your ears.
- If you also are taking an antacid, do not take it within 2 hours of ciprofloxacin or levofloxacin.

Possible Side Effects

Upset stomach, diarrhea, nausea, vomiting, low blood sugar

Antifungal Medications

Antifungal medications are prescribed to prevent and treat infections that are caused by fungus or yeast. These include infections in the mouth (also called **thrush**), vagina (yeast infections), skin (jock itch, athlete's foot), blood, or lungs. There are several commonly prescribed antifungal medicines, including mycostatin, clotrimazole, ketoconazole, and fluconazole.

Thrush
a fungal infection in the mouth.

Mycostatin (nystatin) is an antifungal medication primarily used to prevent thrush from developing in the mouth. It also comes in a powder to treat fungal skin infections like athlete's foot.

Notes about Mycostatin

- Mycostatin is a mouthwash that prevents or treats infections in your mouth.
- Mycostatin should be taken after meals and at bedtime.
- Make sure you do not have anything in your mouth before taking mycostatin.
- Mycostatin is swished around in your mouth for a few minutes and then is swallowed.
- You should not eat or drink anything for 15 to 20 minutes after taking this medicine.
- Take good care of your mouth by brushing and flossing your teeth regularly.

Possible Side Effects

Nausea

Clotrimazole (Mycelex) is an alternative to mycostatin to prevent thrush.

Medications

Notes about Clotrimazole

- Clotrimazole is a lozenge that prevents or treats mouth infections.
- Clotrimazole should be taken after meals and at bedtime.
- You should let the lozenge dissolve in your mouth over a period of 15 minutes.
- Do not chew the lozenges or swallow them whole.

Possible Side Effects

Nausea, vomiting

Ketoconazole (Nizoral) is another antifungal medication.

Notes about Ketoconazole

- Ketoconazole is a pill that should always be taken with food.
- Do not drink alcoholic beverages when taking ketoconazole.
- Antacids and acid blockers, such as Pepcid, Tagamet, or Zantac, should not be taken for at least 2 hours after taking ketoconazole.
- Call your doctor if you have a rash, itching, dark urine, pale stools, yellow skin, or sores in your mouth.
- Ketoconazole can affect the levels of cyclosporine or tacrolimus found in your blood.
- Do not stop taking ketoconazole or change the dose or the time at which you take it unless your transplant team instructs you to do so, because such a change could have a serious effect on your cyclosporine or tacrolimus blood levels.

Possible Side Effects

Diarrhea, nausea, vomiting, impotence, menstrual irregularity, dizziness

Fluconazole (Diflucan) is an antifungal with many uses. It can be used to treat known fungal infections and is often prescribed to prevent fungal infections.

Notes about Fluconazole

- Fluconazole can affect the amount of cyclosporine or tacrolimus found in your blood.
- Do not stop taking fluconazole or change the dose or the time at which you take it unless your transplant team instructs you to do so, because such a change could have a serious effect on your cyclosporine or tacrolimus blood levels.

Possible Side Effects

Nausea, vomiting, diarrhea

Antiviral Medications

Antiviral medications are prescribed to reduce the chance of specific viral infections, such as CMV and herpes, occurring after your transplant. You are at risk of developing these infections if you or your donor have had them at any time before transplantation. Antiviral medicines include valganciclovir, ganciclovir, and acyclovir.

Valganciclovir (Valcyte) and **ganciclovir** (Cytovene) are antiviral agents effective against the herpes viruses. These viruses include herpes simplex, CMV, and varicella (chickenpox).

Notes about Valganciclovir and Ganciclovir

- Do not stop taking valganciclovir or ganciclovir or change the dose or the time at which you take it unless your transplant team instructs you to do so.
- Valganciclovir and ganciclovir can be given in pill form or intravenously (in the vein).
- Call your transplant team if you have a skin rash, sore throat, fever, chills, or pain.

Possible Side Effects

Fever, rash, headache, abnormal kidney function tests, increased risk of infection, fatigue, diarrhea, nausea, vomiting

Acyclovir (Zovirax) is occasionally used to prevent or treat herpes infections or varicella.

Notes about Acyclovir

- Do not become pregnant or father a child while you are taking acyclovir.
- Do not stop taking acyclovir or change the dose or the time at which you take it unless your transplant team instructs you to do so.
- If you are taking acyclovir for herpes simplex infection of the mouth or genitals, avoid kissing and sex if you have open sores.

Possible Side Effects

Nausea, vomiting, diarrhea, abnormal kidney function tests, rash, headache

Medicines That Protect Your Digestive System

Two types of medicines that protect your digestive system are acid blockers and antacids. These agents are often necessary after transplantation to prevent stress ulcers in the stomach and gastroesophageal reflux disease or heartburn symptoms.

Histamine-2 (H$_2$) acid blockers decrease the amount of acid produced by your stomach. They are used to prevent and treat ulcers. The most commonly used H$_2$ acid blockers are **cimetidine** (Tagamet), **ranitidine** (Zantac), **famotidine** (Pepcid), and **nizatidine** (Axid). These drugs are now available over the counter but your transplant physician may want you to take prescription-strength doses.

Notes about Histamine-2 Acid Blockers

- Do not take an acid blocker at the same time you take fluconazole, ketoconazole, or another antacid.
- Take your acid blocker before meals.
- Your doctor will prescribe an acid blocker based on your needs.

Possible Side Effects

Diarrhea, constipation, nausea, gas, headache, dizziness

Proton pump inhibitors block the formation of gastric acid in the stomach by inhibiting the activity at the surface where secretions are produced. The most commonly used proton pump inhibitors are **omeprazole**

(Prilosec), **lansoprazole** (Prevacid), **esomeprozole** (Nexium), **pantoprazole** (Protonix), and **rabeprazole** (Aciphex). They are very well tolerated and extremely effective in treating ulcers and heartburn.

Notes about Proton Pump Inhibitors

- Swallow capsules whole. Do not open or crush them.

Possible Side Effects

Headache, diarrhea, abdominal pain

High Blood Pressure Medications (Antihypertensives)

People who take high blood pressure medications before surgery are likely to continue to need those medications to lower their blood pressure after surgery. In addition, some people who had normal blood pressure before surgery may have high blood pressure after a transplant. Both cyclosporine and tacrolimus cause hypertension in about 70 percent of people who take them. The most commonly prescribed medicines for high blood pressure include **diltiazem** (Cardizem, Cartia, Dilacor, Tiazac), **enalapril** (Vasotec), **lisinopril** (Zestril), **nifedipine** (Procardia, Adalat), **atenolol** (Tenormin), **metoprolol** (Lopressor), and **captopril** (Capoten).

Notes about Antihypertensive Medications

- You may be advised to follow a low-sodium diet if you have or develop high blood pressure.

- Some high blood pressure medications can affect your cyclosporine or tacrolimus blood levels. Check with your transplant team before starting or stopping any high blood pressure medication.

Possible Side Effects

Dizziness and light-headedness for the first few days, fatigue, nausea, loss of appetite, headache, rash, dry cough, swelling in the feet, slow pulse, high potassium levels, kidney dysfunction

Low Blood Pressure Medications

If your blood pressure is too low, your doctor may prescribe medicine to raise it. The medicine most commonly prescribed for low blood pressure is **fludrocortisone** (Florinef).

Notes about Fludrocortisone

- Fludrocortisone raises blood pressure by helping you to retain salt in your body and to discard potassium in your urine.
- Mild ankle swelling is common.
- Fludrocortisone usually is taken in the morning.
- Take fludrocortisone under close medical supervision.

Possible Side Effects

Swelling in the hands or feet, rapid weight gain, water retention, headache

Diuretics

Patients who take prednisone may retain excess fluid in their bodies. Removing excess fluid also is helpful for lowering blood pressure. Diuretic medications (fluid pills) may be used briefly after transplantation to help you get rid of excess fluids caused by intravenous hydration during the surgery and while you were unable to eat. The most commonly used diuretics are **furosemide** (Lasix), **hydrochlorothiazide** (HCTZ), **torsemide** (Demadex), and **bumetanide** (Bumex). **Spironolactone** (Aldactone) may have been one of your diuretics before transplantation—this medication should *not* be used after transplantation.

Notes about Diuretics

- Take the diuretic early in the day so that you will not have to get up several times a night to go to the bathroom.
- Taking a diuretic could cause your body to lose potassium. Potassium supplements may be prescribed for a short time to replenish the supply in your blood.
- Do not increase or decrease the dosage of your diuretic without consulting your transplant team.

Possible Side Effects

Low blood pressure, dizziness, light-headedness, dehydration, more frequent urination, low potassium

Cholesterol-Lowering Medications

Lowering your cholesterol may help prevent heart disease. People who have high cholesterol levels may be given medicine to lower it. The primary immunosuppressive agents cyclosporine and sirolimus often cause high cholesterol and triglyceride levels in many patients who take them. The most commonly used cholesterol-lowering medicines are **atorvastatin** (Lipitor), **simvastatin** (Zocor), **pravastatin** (Pravachol), and **lovastatin** (Mevacor).

Notes about Cholesterol-Lowering Medications

- Cholesterol-lowering medicines usually are taken at night.
- The results of taking a cholesterol-lowering medication may not be seen for weeks or months.
- You will have blood tests while taking a cholesterol-lowering medicine to confirm that your liver is functioning normally and to monitor your cholesterol levels.
- Do not take a cholesterol-lowering medication if you are pregnant or considering pregnancy.
- Call the doctor who prescribed the cholesterol-lowering medication immediately if you experience muscle cramps or weakness, especially in your legs.

Possible Side Effects

Upset stomach, heartburn, change in the way foods taste, diarrhea, skin rash, headache, constipation, blurred vision, muscle damage

Drug Interactions

Some medicines can interfere with the way cyclosporine, tacrolimus, and sirolimus are processed in your body and can lead to very high or very low blood levels of these drugs. This effect can result in toxicity or rejection of the transplanted liver. Be sure to discuss possible drug interactions with any physician who prescribes a new medicine for you. If you are unsure about a new medication, contact your transplant team.

PART NINE

Complications

What is acute rejection?

Now that I am immunosuppressed, am I
susceptible to infections?

What is chronic rejection?

More...

79. What is acute rejection?

Rejection is a signal that your immune system has identified your new liver as foreign tissue and is trying to get rid of it. Preventing rejection with immunosuppressive medications is the first priority. An episode of rejection of the transplanted liver is very common, occurring in as many as 60 percent of liver recipients. Most people experience a rejection episode within 5 to 10 days of the transplant operation. The signs you and your doctors and nurses are watching for include a low-grade temperature, decreased appetite, abdominal discomfort, joint and/or back pain, tenderness over the liver, increased abdominal fluid, and feeling like you might have the flu. Other signs include an elevation of your liver function blood tests, a change in the color of your bile (from dark green to light yellow), and a decrease in the amount of bile produced.

An episode of rejection of the transplanted liver is very common, occurring in as many as 60 percent of liver recipients.

Because most people do not have obvious signs of rejection, your liver function tests will be monitored closely. If they are abnormal, a liver biopsy may be performed to confirm that you are experiencing a rejection episode. A liver biopsy is accomplished at the hospital bedside. The upper part of your incision is closed by staples, which are removed several days after your surgery. This permits access to the new liver by a biopsy needle. A liver biopsy usually is not painful, but you will feel pressure when the needle is inserted into the liver. Liver biopsies also can be performed on an outpatient basis. This procedure may be necessary if your liver function tests rise after you go home from the hospital.

If you have an episode of rejection, the amount of anti-rejection medication you are taking will be increased, or a different combination of anti-rejection medications will be prescribed. In almost all cases, *adjusting the medications will stop the rejection episode.*

80. Now that I am immunosuppressed, am I susceptible to infections?

The anti-rejection medications that you are taking to prevent and treat rejection tell your immune system to accept your new liver. In doing so, they may also tell your immune system to accept other foreign invaders that it ordinarily would fight. As a consequence, taking anti-rejection medications can place you at greater risk for developing an infection. The most common infections result from viruses that have been lying dormant in your system or in the donated liver. To prevent infection, you will take antibacterial, antivirus, and antifungal medications for 3 to 6 months after your surgery.

If an infection is suspected, your caregivers may take sputum (the substance coughed up from your lungs), blood, and urine samples, as well as samples from your catheter, wound, and drain sites. Signs that you may notice include fever; tiredness or fatigue; diarrhea or vomiting; redness or drainage around your incision, bile, or tube site; or a cough and sore throat. If an infection develops, it will be treated with medication specific for the type of infection. The infectious disease specialist works with the transplant team to manage and treat infections. If an infection develops after you have been discharged from the hospital, it may be treated with antibiotics on an outpatient basis. However, some people need to be readmitted to the hospital for treatment with intravenous medications.

81. What is chronic rejection?

Chronic rejection (CR) involves progressive deterioration of the transplanted liver's function. It is thought to be caused by immune reactivity leading to scarring of the liver. The targets of the **immune response** are different from the targets in acute rejection. In CR, the arteries and bile ducts are most likely to be affected and damaged. This damage occurs very slowly and is not a result of recurrent episodes of acute rejection. CR may be exacerbated by factors such as cytomegalovirus infection, high cholesterol levels, diabetes, or hypertension.

Chronic liver rejection is uncommon but is most likely due to the unique immunologic properties of the liver **allograft**, the regenerative capacity of the liver, and our ability to better recognize and control acute rejection. The main cause of CR, as with acute rejection, is too little immunosuppressive medication—either because the patient does not take his or her medications as prescribed or because the transplant physician reduces the dose in an attempt to avoid side effects. CR occurs in only 1 to 3 percent of transplantation cases, however. Chronic liver rejection was once thought to indicate the need for retransplantation. However, thanks to our earlier recognition of acute and chronic rejection and the introduction of more powerful immunosuppressive agents (for example, tacrolimus and sirolimus), many of these cases can be successfully reversed.

82. What is a liver biopsy?

Blood tests, ultrasounds, and computer tomography scans may all provide information about the status of your liver. Nevertheless, sometimes looking at actual liver tissue becomes necessary. For example, recurrent

Immune response

a defensive action by the immune system.

Allograft

a graft between two individuals who are of the same species (e.g., human) but have genetic differences.

hepatitis C rejection and CR can be diagnosed only by examining liver tissue under a microscope. In these cases, a liver biopsy is performed. This procedure can provide critical information about the cause and extent of a patient's liver disease, and it will allow the transplant physician to choose the appropriate treatment.

For example, in recurrent hepatitis C, the liver enzyme tests (**AST** and **ALT**) may be normal or elevated. In such a case, a liver biopsy must be performed to assess the actual degree of damage to the liver. If there is active inflammation or scarring, you may need treatment to eradicate or control the hepatitis C virus.

AST

aspartate amino-transferase; a type of liver enzyme.

ALT

alanine aminotrans-ferase; a type of liver enzyme.

Many staging systems for interpreting a liver biopsy have been developed. The most commonly used system assigns a number between 0 and 4 for the amount of inflammation in the liver and a number between 0 and 4 for the amount of scarring in the liver. The inflammation number is termed the grade, and the scarring number is termed the stage. A stage 0 biopsy is normal, whereas a stage 4 biopsy has enough scarring to be classified as cirrhosis. Stages 1, 2, and 3 represent steps between stage 0 and stage 4 (cirrhosis). Similarly, grade 0 means no inflammation. Grade 1 indicates minimal inflammation, grade 2 means mild inflammation, grade 3 means moderate inflammation, and grade 4 is severe inflammation. The pathologist will also comment on other features such as where the inflammation is located and whether rejection is evident in the biopsy specimen.

If you are asked to undergo a liver biopsy, you will have blood tests first to ensure you do not have an increased risk of bleeding after the procedure. In addition, if there is time, you should discontinue aspirin and aspirin-like products (such as ibuprofen) 3 to 7 days before the biopsy. You should not eat any food on the day of your biopsy. Your doctor or a member of the radiology department may perform the biopsy (see Figure 8). Initially, your skin will be cleaned with a solution to reduce the risk of infection. Then, the skin is numbed by injection with a medication called lidocaine. Often, an ultrasound device is used to guide the procedure. A biopsy needle is rapidly inserted about 1 inch into the liver and removed. A sample of tissue (only 1/50,000th of your liver!) is removed through the needle and sent to the pathology department for further processing.

The biopsy may be performed on an inpatient or outpatient basis. Although it takes less than a half-hour, you may be monitored for several hours after the procedure. The results are usually available within 24 hours.

The most common complication of a liver biopsy is pain. This discomfort usually takes the form of a dull ache in the right upper abdomen or shoulder and typically resolves within 2 hours with or without pain medications. Bleeding, infection, and drug reactions are other less common but potentially serious complications of a biopsy. Unrelenting pain is rare and could indicate a severe complication—you should notify your doctor immediately if this occurs.

The success of liver transplantation has resulted in longer survival after the operation for today's patients.

83. Do I have to worry about long-term effects of immunosuppression?

The success of liver transplantation has resulted in longer survival after the operation for today's patients. This longer survival comes at a price, however: far more long-term complications than were seen in the past. More attention must therefore be paid to the long-term effects of the immunosuppressive drugs and their cumulative effects. For example, cyclosporine can cause hypertension and high cholesterol. Over the course of many years, this combination results in heart attack and stroke. When expected survival after transplantation was short, these long-term issues were of minimal concern. Today, with longer survival being commonplace, heart disease is one of the major causes of death in transplant recipients.

The incidence of hypertension—estimated at 50 to 65 percent after liver transplantation—is attributed to the primary immunosuppressive agents. Standard antihypertensive medications are effective in treating this complication. As noted earlier, over the long term hypertension can result in heart or vascular disease.

Obesity is another common problem after transplantation. Because many patients suffer from malnutrition prior to transplantation, these individuals are counseled to improve their nutrition afterward to help the healing process. Unfortunately, patients may become accustomed to this increased calorie intake and have a hard time cutting back their food consumption once recovery from surgery has been achieved. The subsequent obesity can decrease mobility and increase the risk of coronary artery disease.

Diabetes mellitus is frequently encountered in liver transplant recipients. Once again, the culprit is often the immunosuppressive agents, particularly tacrolimus and prednisone. The incidence of obesity correlates with diabetes incidence, and both are cardiac risk factors.

Transplant-associated lymphoma is a feared complication of the immunosuppressive drugs. Fortunately, it occurs in only 1 to 2 percent of transplant recipients. This kind of lymphoma is associated with the use of OKT3 and infection with the Epstein-Barr virus. Many patients who develop post-transplant lymphoproliferative disease (PTLD) can be treated with a reduction in immunosuppression, which may cause the PTLD to regress. In rare cases, the PTLD becomes a true lymphoma and chemotherapy is required.

Transplant recipients have higher rates of both skin cancer and cervical cancer. Proper skin care, especially sun protection, is essential in these patients. For women, annual Pap smears are recommended.

84. I've heard that I might develop kidney problems after liver transplantation. How can that happen?

Chronic renal failure is a recognized complication of all organ transplantation due to the need for immunosuppression. Both tacrolimus and cyclosporine can cause the kidneys to function less than optimally. Additionally, in patients with cirrhosis, renal disease before transplantation, the side effects of diuretic use, hypertension, and diabetes can all contribute to chronic renal failure in recipients of a new liver. Renal failure after the transplantation of the liver complicates medical management, leading to increased morbidity and mortality. The incidence of chronic renal disease among recipients of liver transplants is approximately 8 percent after 1 year, 12 percent after 2 years, and 18 percent after 3 years. This does not mean that all of

Chronic renal failure

when kidneys slowly lose function over a period of time and do not regain their function. This condition requires long-term dialysis or transplantation.

these patients need dialysis but rather that their kidneys are not fully functional. Some patients do, indeed, progress to dialysis; kidney transplantation may be indicated in these individuals.

A number of factors may predict the risk of developing renal failure, including age (older patients have a higher risk); gender (males have a higher risk than females); pre-transplantation kidney function; and presence or absence of pre-transplantation hypertension, diabetes, or hepatitis C infection. Overall, non-Caucasian, non-African American patients have the lowest risk of chronic renal failure.

Of course, most liver transplant recipients do *not* develop renal failure. For those with the risk factors mentioned previously, transplant physicians can work with them to reduce the risk of developing renal failure after liver transplantation. One technique is to reduce the dose of the primary immunosuppressive agent (that is, tacrolimus or cyclosporine). For those patients with a high risk or history of rejection, mycophenolate mofetil (CellCept) or mycophenolate sodium (Myfortic) can be added to the drug regimen. A recent addition to the immunosuppression armamentarium, sirolimus (Rapamycin, Rapamune), can also reduce the risk. Sirolimus is not toxic to the kidneys and may be used for primary immunosuppression. This drug cannot be used immediately after liver transplantation because it slows wound healing; instead, it is typically prescribed later if concerns about renal dysfunction arise.

PART TEN

Living Donor Liver Transplantation

What is the difference between the right and left lobes of the liver?

What is a living donor liver transplant?

What is a split donor liver transplant?

More...

85. What is the difference between the right and left lobes of the liver?

The liver is actually divided into three lobes: right, left, and caudate (Figure 9). The caudate lobe, which is usually very small, is located behind the right lobe. All three lobes of the liver are made up of the same tissue: liver cells, blood vessels, and bile ducts. They have the same functions and ability to regenerate (grow in size). The right lobe is larger, often accounting for 60 to 70 percent of the liver. Because both lobes are the same and have the ability to grow, either can be removed. The remaining lobe will regenerate by increasing in size. Thus, for example, the liver will not "regrow" a new right lobe if the right lobe has been removed surgically. Instead, the whole liver will be an enlarged left lobe. After removal of a lobe, the liver functions nor-

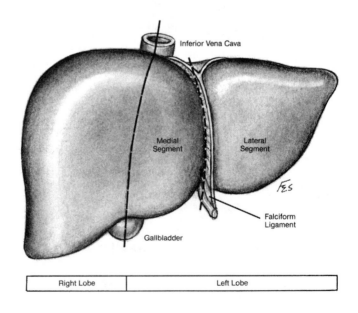

Figure 9   Liver Anatomy. Illustration courtesy of Roger Jenkins, MD, who holds the rights.

mally almost immediately. This allows transplant surgeons to remove a full lobe and transplant it into another person in need of liver transplantation.

86. What is a living donor liver transplant?

The unique anatomy of the liver allows it to be separated into independent anatomical units that are able to retain their normal function (Figure 10). Since 1989, several thousand living donor liver transplant (LDLT) operations have been performed worldwide, most commonly between an adult donor and a pediatric recipient. These procedures have significantly reduced the number of pediatric patients who die while on the waiting list.

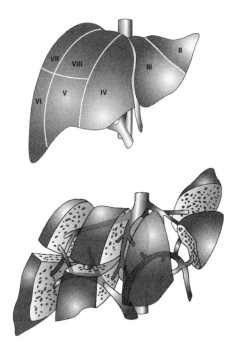

Figure 10   Liver Segments. Reprinted with permission from Memorial Sloan-Kettering.

Current data suggest that the results of LDLTs are at least similar to, and perhaps better than, the results of cadaveric liver transplants. Because it can potentially increase the number of people who may benefit from liver transplantation, LDLT poses exciting, new surgical possibilities for adult patients with end-stage liver disease. The basis for taking part of a living person's liver lies in a healthy liver's unique ability to grow back or regenerate to normal size for both the donor and the recipient.

The basis for taking part of a living person's liver lies in a healthy liver's unique ability to grow back or regenerate to normal size for both the donor and the recipient.

In these highly technical operations, the right lobe of the donor's liver (about 60 percent of the total liver) is implanted into the recipient. The recipient's entire liver is removed because it is diseased and functions poorly. Following surgery, the rapid regeneration of the liver allows both the donor's and the recipient's livers to return to nearly full size. Amazingly, it typically takes the recipient's liver less than 1 month to regenerate fully. That time frame is a bit longer for the donor, whose liver will often take a full year to accomplish the same feat.

Because the left lobe is the smaller of the two lobes, it can be used as a living donor organ only in children or very small adults. The larger right lobe is needed when the recipient is an average-size or larger adult.

Jonathan's comments:

I have many wonderful people in my life with whom I have shared many rich and meaningful experiences. When a person is willing to put himself or herself in harm's way by donating a lobe of his or her liver so that you can survive, it is an amazingly powerful experience. Words cannot describe the bond and connection created when a person gives you a part of himself or herself. My sister and I have a bond like no other people in our lives, and I will be forever grateful to her.

87. What is a split donor liver transplant?

A split donor liver transplant is different from an LDLT. In the living donor transplant, the healthy donor gives up one lobe (usually the right) and keeps the smaller lobe. Both lobes then regenerate to nearly normal size. In this kind of surgery, no cadaveric organs are used to transplant the recipient.

In a split donor transplant, an adult cadaveric organ is divided into the left and right lobes. The left lobe is often transplanted into a child, and the right lobe is placed into an adult from the waiting list. The split liver transplant therefore benefits the pediatric patients on the waiting list, because an adult organ is used as a transplant in a child. The use of split livers has virtually eliminated any waiting time for pediatric livers because adult donors are far more common than pediatric donors. The adults on the waiting list, however, do not gain an "extra" organ because only one adult will be transplanted from the adult cadaver donor.

88. Why is living donor transplantation necessary?

Liver transplantation remains the best treatment for people with end-stage liver disease; however, only enough organs from brain-dead donors become available to help one-third of the more than 17,000 people on the United Network for Organ Sharing (UNOS) liver transplant waiting list. Sadly, about 20 percent of patients die each year while waiting for a suitable liver. This scarcity of donors has driven medical professionals to explore what would otherwise be considered an extreme solution to liver failure—living donor liver transplantation.

Although LDLT will never replace traditional deceased donor transplantation, it may offer the possibility of liver transplantation to an additional 20 to 40 percent of patients on the UNOS waiting list. The immediate benefits of LDLT are twofold. First, because LDLT is an elective procedure performed when the recipient is in the "best" condition, he or she avoids the continued physical deterioration that inevitably occurs while waiting for a suitable liver replacement. Second, by avoiding the use of a deceased donor liver, LDLT helps to shorten the UNOS waiting list and allows another patient on that list to benefit from transplantation.

Jonathan's comments:

As it turned out, my condition became so critical in such a short period of time that a cadaver liver was not a option. In retrospect, my condition was worse than my MELD score indicated. Chances are very likely I would have died while waiting for a cadaver liver. A live donor transplant was my only option, and my sister was a perfect match.

89. Who can be a donor?

A potential donor must first volunteer to donate a portion of his or her liver to a family member or someone with whom he or she shares strong emotional ties. Not all volunteers, however, are deemed suitable. The donor's blood type must be compatible with the recipient's blood type (see Table 4), and his or her liver must be large enough relative to the recipient's body size.

Many living donor transplant centers also enforce age and weight limitations. Typically, donors must be at least 18 years of age. This not only increases the likelihood of an adequate donor liver size but also ensures that the donor is of legal age to consent to the procedure. It would certainly be awkward—if not unethical—for a cirrhotic parent to consent to both his or her own operation and the donor's operation if the donor was under 18 years of age. Careful screening tests must be performed to evaluate the health and suitability of the donor. These tests include basic laboratory tests, a full medical evaluation, and imaging (computer tomography [CT] scan or magnetic resonance imaging) of the liver to determine the size of each lobe and the vascular (blood vessel) anatomy.

The decision to donate part of one's liver can be extremely difficult. By definition, the donor is healthy and, therefore, does not need major abdominal surgery and its attendant risks. Many factors must be considered in this decision, including the medical issues mentioned previously. Does the donor have something to gain from the operation—specifically, more quality time with the healthy recipient? How would the donor feel about the surgery if he or she developed a complication? What if the recipient had a complication or died? Psychiatric evaluations are conducted to ensure that the donor does not feel unduly pressured by other family members and is truly willing to undergo the procedure.

90. What are the risks and benefits to the donor?

As with any surgical procedure, there are risks involved in donating a part of the liver. Living donors receive general anesthesia for the operation, and LDLT is considered major surgery. All patients experience some discomfort and pain after an operation. Living donors may develop complications such as infections, bleeding, or even death.

Although most donors report an overall positive experience, it is possible to have negative psychological consequences from such a donation. There may be pressure from family members or even from themselves to donate. If there is any ambivalence on the donor's part, he or she may feel guilty. If the donor evaluation determines that the potential donor is not suitable, feelings of resentment from the recipient or his family may arise. Similar feelings may occur if, after donation, the recipient has an episode of rejection. It is important that potential donors, recipients, and their families be aware of these issues and have adequate support available if any occur. These supports come from the transplant team, mental health professionals, and close friends and family.

Of course, there are also many positive aspects to living donation. Although donating a part of the liver offers no direct medical benefit for the donor, it has significant advantages for the recipient. The surgery can be scheduled at a time when the recipient is in fairly good physical condition (timing is very important—the recipient should neither be too sick nor too well). Because LDLT is an elective operation, the surgery can be scheduled at a time that is convenient for both the donor and the recipient. A living donor transplant shortens the length of time the recipient must wait for an organ, usually shortens the hospital stay, and eliminates the stressful period of waiting for a suitable organ to become available.

Living donation also offers the donor and the recipient more time together, once the recipient becomes healthy again. This extra time will enhance both parties' lives. The recipient can experience positive feelings, knowing that the gift came from a loved one. The donor can be comforted, knowing that he or she has helped not only a loved one but also another person on the waiting list, who can now receive a cadaveric organ that might have otherwise gone to the living donor recipient.

Jonathan's comments:

When my sister offered to donate a lobe of her liver, I was thrilled, but at the same time frightened for her. All the way up to the last few moments before they took us both in for the surgery, I told her it was okay if she changed her mind. I wanted her to feel as comfortable as she could about her decision knowing it was a highly [emotionally charged] situation. A response she gave that I will never forget was "The best thing that could happen is that we do this and get your life back." My sister's commitment to carrying through with her decision was another source of inspiration to carry me through this ordeal.

91. What is the evaluation process for the donor?

After initial screening blood work is received and reviewed, a potential donor is scheduled for a consult with a transplant nurse and a surgeon. This consult involves a discussion of the procedure itself and gives the donor an opportunity to ask any questions.

The potential donor is then scheduled, along with the recipient, for a CT scan or MRI to evaluate liver volume and vascular anatomy. More extensive blood work is also completed at this time.

If the donor is accepted based on his or her liver anatomy, a comprehensive medical and psychosocial evaluation is then scheduled. This evaluation includes an ultrasound, preoperative testing, and consults with a physician, psychiatrist, and social worker. If a potential donor completes this evaluation successfully and is accepted as a suitable donor, surgery is scheduled.

The process of living donor evaluation usually takes several days or weeks. It is necessary to search for all issues that might potentially affect the surgery or the successful recovery of the donor. It is also important to give the donor adequate time to reflect on his or her decision to donate. Liver donation is a major decision that affects not only the lives of the recipient and the donor but also the lives of their families. Some potential donors step forward with good intentions but, during the evaluation process, learn about the risks and benefits that were not known prior to volunteering. This may result in ambivalence about the procedure. It may be difficult for a potential donor who is already well into the evaluation to stop the process if it is moving along too quickly. For this reason, a slow and steady evaluation, with donor advocates who are not members of the transplant team per se, and the ability for anyone involved in the process to call off the surgery at any time without fear of penalty or loss of dignity or privacy are mandatory.

92. Who pays for the donor?

The donor's evaluation and operation expenses are usually covered by insurance. The transplant program will first check with the donor's health insurance company to see if it has a policy regarding coverage for organ donation. Many companies do, indeed, have a policy in place stating that they will (or will not) cover the evaluation and operation. If the donor's health insurance does not provide payment, the recipient's insurance company is contacted. Typically, the recipient's health insurance pays for all of the donor and recipient evaluations and operations.

Coverage for donor complications from surgery is far more variable. Some donors' insurance companies will readily pay for any complication; others will not. Although complications are not common, the donor must investigate and prepare for this possibility in case it becomes reality. The transplant team's financial coordinator can help guide the donor through this process.

93. How is the surgery performed, and how long will it take?

Two separate surgical teams perform the donor and recipient surgeries simultaneously. As one team works on removing the diseased liver from the recipient, the other team focuses on removing a portion of the donor's healthy liver. Typically, the right lobe of the donor's liver is removed, which accounts for approximately 60 percent of total liver volume.

The operation to remove the right lobe is called a liver resection. After the donor is put to sleep with anesthesia, an incision is made across the upper abdomen underneath the rib cage. This incision is 8 to 12 inches long. The piece of liver is removed and prepared to be transplanted into the recipient. While the liver is being prepared for and then transplanted to the recipient (who is in an adjacent operating room), the donor's incision is closed and stitched. After the surgery, the donor is moved to the recovery room (post-anesthesia care unit) and monitored closely. In fact, some donors stay in the post-anesthesia care unit overnight. The donor surgery typically takes about 6 hours, and the recipient surgery about 5 hours.

94. Could the donor die?

Yes, there is an extremely small risk of donor death due to the operation. This risk is estimated to be less than 0.2 percent, or 1 in 500. To date, there have been 3 deaths reported in adult right lobe liver donors in the United States. Additionally, one living donor required transplantation soon after donation. There were no known similarities in the donors who died.

95. How long is the donor in the hospital? Out of work?

The average donor will be in the hospital for 7 to 10 days and will need to stay near the transplant program for approximately 1 week following discharge. The donor can recover at home but will need some assistance from friends and family as he or she recuperates from this major abdominal surgery. During the first few weeks after the surgery, the donor will be able to accomplish many of the activities of normal living but will need help performing tasks that require lifting more than 5 pounds. Activity can be gradually increased over the next few weeks. The donor is typically out of work for 6 to 12 weeks depending on the type of work he or she does. For example, donors with sedentary jobs may be able to return to work at least part-time in 6 to 8 weeks. Donors who perform manual labor usually need 8 to 12 weeks to recover.

Much like the recipient, the donor can expect some indirect expenses related to the evaluation and hospitalization. The donor's—or, more likely, the recipient's—health insurance will cover the donor's tests and physician and hospital expenses. Insurance companies rarely pay for the donor's transportation costs, food, lodging, child care expenses, or lost wages. Additional sources of funding, such as savings accounts, fundraisers, and the recipient, may be necessary to cover these costs. Coverage for post-donation complications vary from one insurance plan to the next and should be investigated prior to donation.

96. Are the results as good if I have a living donor compared to a cadaver donor?

Cadaveric liver transplantation has been the standard of care for patients with liver failure for more than 20 years. Hence over time many transplant surgeons and programs have developed the skills and structure necessary to perform this operation successfully. This includes the ability to accept and list the most appropriate candidates, perform the surgery, assist in the recipient's recovery, and provide the necessary postoperative care and support. As a consequence, there is the expectation of excellent outcomes from cadaveric liver transplantation.

In the past 5 years, living donor liver transplantation programs have been developed at hospitals with the goal of expanding the donor pool. Early reports showed that living donor recipients' outcomes were not as good as the outcomes experienced by their cadaver recipient counterparts. Later reports from LDLT programs with the most experience have now shown that LDLT can have at least equal, if not superior, outcomes. This increased effectiveness is likely attributable to the same factors that made cadaveric donor transplantation successful 20 years ago—experience in selecting appropriate recipients and donors, evolving surgical skill, and the infrastructure to optimize outcomes for all.

Later reports from LDLT programs with the most experience have now shown that LDLT can have at least equal, if not superior, outcomes.

In addition, LDLT enjoys some other potential benefits over cadaver donor transplantation. First, recipients may have an opportunity to undergo transplantation long before life-threatening liver-related events occur. They are likely to be in better physical and nutritional shape than patients awaiting cadaver donations. Second, the living donor liver, although smaller in size than a cadaveric liver, is more likely to have "ideal donor" (see Question 20) characteristics. Third, the medical cost of the year prior to transplantation has been estimated to be approximately $100,000. By undergoing transplantation earlier in the course of the disease, much of this money can be saved. Lastly, the use of living donor livers results in more cadaver livers for patients in need of transplantation who do not have the option of LDLT. In some ways, a living donor transplant may save two lives.

97. If I have a relative donate part of his or her liver to me, do I need to take immunosuppressive drugs? Does the donor?

After undergoing an LDLT, the recipient will still need to take the standard drugs necessary to prevent rejection. Unless the organ is donated by the recipient's identical twin, there remain many genetic dissimilarities between the original and donated organs. As a consequence, rejection is a lifelong concern, just as it would be in a cadaveric donor liver transplant.

The donor does not have to take any special medication to prevent rejection because the regenerated liver will be his or her own. The donor's body and immune system will recognize the regenerated liver as its own, so there is no risk of rejection.

98. My brother was rejected as a recipient candidate at our local transplant program. Will they reconsider him if I donate part of my liver?

Most programs that perform LDLT have been performing cadaveric donor liver transplantation for many years. The program is likely to be very experienced in the recipient evaluation process and the reasons for candidate acceptance and rejection. This experience includes an understanding of what makes a liver transplant successful. This understanding is integrated into the acceptance/rejection process.

The criteria for acceptance as a living donor transplant candidate do not differ from those criteria necessary to undergo cadaveric transplantation. The candidate must still (1) meet all of the acceptance standards put forth by the program and (2) have none of the exclusion criteria. The source of the liver for transplantation should not influence the expectations for the candidate's successful surgery, recovery, and long-term health. Therefore, most programs will require the candidate to be accepted for transplantation based on accepted criteria and listed for transplantation with UNOS before considering whether that person could be a living donor recipient. The ability to supply a liver (via living donor) would not make a candidate more acceptable.

99. What does the future hold for liver transplantation?

There are several areas within the field of liver transplantation that are actively evolving.

In the past decade, our knowledge about immunosuppression has increased dramatically. We are becoming more comfortable with the process of recognizing and treating rejection. These advances have allowed transplant physicians to progressively minimize immunosuppression, using just enough medications to prevent rejection while simultaneously decreasing the side effects and risks associated with the drugs. Several new medications have become available that are associated with fewer side effects—sirolimus, for example, does not cause renal insufficiency like the other primary agents. There are other agents currently in development, all of which aim to provide adequate anti-rejection properties without the risks linked to the current medications. Scientists and transplant clinicians are also experimenting with ways to permanently alter the transplant recipient's immune system so that the transplanted organ is not identified as foreign tissue.

Because of the extreme shortage in donor livers in the United States, much attention has focused on increasing the donor pool. Living donor, split liver, and deceased due to cardiac death donor transplantations are becoming more commonplace. The use of extended criteria donors and hepatitis C–infected donors is also increasing the number of livers available for donation. The optimal use of these nonstandard donor livers and the matching of these livers to the best possible recipients remain goals of organ allocation research. The use of animal livers (known as **xenotransplantation**) is likely years, if not decades, away.

Perhaps most important is research directed toward preserving liver function prior to transplantation. If we can keep native livers functioning adequately, then the need for organ transplantation will diminish dramatically. Increasing the public awareness of high-risk behaviors, such as intravenous drug use and alcohol abuse, is essential. Early recognition of liver disease and development and application of effective treatments are equally important. There is active research looking at the factors that allow the liver to regenerate—perhaps one day these factors can be administered to failing livers.

Research in each of these areas will yield advances over the coming years with the ultimate goal of reduced need for transplantation, improved organ allocation, and more effective management of those who require liver transplantation.

100. Where can I learn more about liver transplantation?

Numerous resources are available to patients with liver disease and their families. You can obtain a wealth of information from your primary care physician, gastroenterologist, hepatologist, or local transplant center. Other resources are available through the Internet. Of course, be aware that the quality of information on the

Xenotrans-plantation

transplantation of an animal organ into a human. Although xenotransplantation is highly experimental, many scientists view it as an eventual solution to the shortage of human organs.

Research in each of these areas will yield advances over the coming years with the ultimate goal of reduced need for transplantation, improved organ allocation, and more effective management of those who require liver transplantation.

177

websites varies widely. Here are some tips to help you evaluate a website:

- Check the "about us" section of the site. If there is no author listed or no credentials for the author, be suspicious.
- Check the attribution of the information. Experts have reviewed research in mainstream journals. Information from major government agencies, such as the Food and Drug Administration and National Institutes of Health, has also been reviewed by experts. Information from drug companies may be reliable but remember—these companies are in the business of selling products.
- Information put out by patient groups can be biased toward one point of view.
- Be wary of emotional testimonials. They can be misleading or irrelevant to you.
- Read many websites and cross-check what you find.
- If a treatment seems too good to be true, it probably is!
- Check with your primary care physician or transplant team before making any changes in your treatment plan based on information you found on the Internet.

Resources

American Liver Foundation
(information, education, support)
75 Maiden Lane, Suite 603
New York, NY 10038-4810
Telephone: 800-223-0179
Website: www.liverfoundation.org

American Organ Transplant Association
(information, education, fundraising information)
3335 Cartwright Road
Missouri City, TX 77459-2548
Telephone: 281-261-2682
E-mail: aota@pdq.net

Centers for Medicare and Medicaid Services
Website: www.cms.hhs.gov

Children's Liver Association for Support Services
Website: www.classkids.org

Department of Public Health
(financial assistance)
Division of Organ Transplant Services
10 West Street
Boston, MA 02111
Telephone: 617-753-8130

Latino Organization for Liver Awareness (LOLA)
(information and education for Spanish-speaking individuals)
1560 Mayflower Avenue
Bronx, NY 10465
Telephone: 718-892-8697

Medicare
Website: www.medicare.gov

National Council on Patient Information and Education (NCPIE)
(consumer's guide, information, education)
666 11th Street NW, Suite 810
Washington, DC 20001
Telephone: 202-347-6711
E-mail: ncple@erols.com

National Digestive Diseases Information Clearinghouse
Website: http://digestive.niddk.nih.gov

National Foundation for Transplants
(fundraising information and short-term financial assistance)
1102 Brookfield Road, Suite 202
Memphis, TN 38119
Telephone: 800-489-3863
E-mail: natfoundtx@aol.com
Website: www.transplants.org

National Institutes of Health
(research trials)
Website: http://clinicaltrials.gov/search/intervention=
  %22liver+transplantation%22&recruiting=true

Scientific Registry of Transplant Recipients
Website: www.ustransplant.org

Transplant Foundation
(fundraising assistance)
8002 Discovery Drive, Suite 310
Richmond, VA 23229
Telephone: 804-285-5115

Transplant Recipients International Organization (TRIO)
(information, education, peer networking, and support)
1000 16th Street, NW, Suite 602
Washington, DC 20036
Telephone: 800-874-6386
Website: www.trioweb.org

United Network for Organ Sharing (UNOS)
Telephone: 888-894-6361
Website: www.unos.org

Resources

Glossary

ABO typing: A blood test to determine blood type. A transplant donor and a recipient must have compatible blood types.

Albumin: A protein made by the liver.

Allograft: A graft between two individuals who are of the same species (e.g., human) but have genetic differences.

ALT: Alanine aminotransferase. See *liver enzymes.*

Anesthesia: Medicine that is given by a specially trained physician or nurse to put a patient to sleep (general anesthesia) or numb an area of the body (local anesthesia) so that a medical procedure or operation can be performed without pain.

Antacid: A medicine that protects the digestive system. It can relieve indigestion and other digestive discomfort.

Antibody: A protein molecule produced by the immune system in response to a foreign body, such as virus or a transplanted organ. Because antibodies fight the transplanted organ and try to reject it, recipients are required to take anti-rejection (immunosuppressive) drugs.

Ascites: Fluid in the abdomen.

AST: Aspartate aminotransferase. See *liver enzymes.*

Bacteria: Small organisms or germs that can cause disease.

Bile: A fluid produced by the liver, stored in the gallbladder, and released into the small intestine to help the body digest fats.

Bile leak: A hole in the bile duct system resulting in bile spilling into the abdomen.

Bile tube: A tube placed in the bile duct that permits bile to drain into a bag outside of the body.

Biliary stenosis: Narrowing or constriction of a bile duct.

Bilirubin: An orange-colored substance in bile that is produced when red blood cells break down.

Biopsy: The procedure during which a piece of tissue is first removed from a part of the body and then examined in the laboratory.

Bladder: The part of the urinary tract that receives urine from the kidneys and stores it until urination.

Brain death: When the brain has permanently stopped working, as determined by a neurological surgeon, artificial support systems may maintain functions such as heartbeat and respiration for a few days.

BUN: Blood urea nitrogen; a waste product (created when proteins break down) excreted by the kidneys. BUN is tested as an indicator of kidney function.

Cadaver: The body of a person who has died.

Cadaveric donor: A recently deceased individual whose death does not affect the quality of his or her organs. The individual and his or her family have agreed to donate organs and tissue for transplantation.

Cardiac: Having to do with the heart.

Cardiologist: A doctor who specializes in diseases of the heart.

Cholesterol: A form of fat that the body needs to perform certain functions. Too much cholesterol can cause heart disease.

Chronic rejection: Slow, continuous immunological attack by the host immune system on the transplanted organ, usually resulting in progressive loss of organ function.

Cirrhosis: Scarring of the liver.

CMV (cytomegalovirus): A virus that lies dormant in the body and can be reactivated after transplantation, causing a flu-like illness, pneumonia, and/or gastrointestinal ulcers.

Creatinine: A substance that is found in blood and urine. Creatinine is measured to determine kidney function.

Criteria (medical criteria): A set of clinical or biologic standards or conditions that must be met.

CT scan: Computerized tomography (computerized axial tomography) scan. A noninvasive x-ray that enables clinicians to see and evaluate internal organs and blood vessels.

Diabetes: A disease in which people are unable to process sugar in the body correctly.

Dialysis: The process by which the blood is cleansed of toxins, and levels of various blood chemicals and fluids are corrected.

Donor: The person who gives an organ to someone else.

Edema: Excess fluid in the tissues of the body. Swollen ankles are a sign of edema.

Electrocardiogram: A recording of the electrical activity of the heart.

Electrolyte: Generally refers to the dissolved form of a mineral such as sodium, potassium, magnesium, or chlorine.

Encephalopathy: A condition often associated with liver disease that is characterized by insomnia, memory loss, and an inability to concentrate or think clearly.

Endoscopy: A procedure performed by a gastroenterologist. After the patient is sedated, a long tube containing a miniaturized camera and bright light is advanced through the mouth into the esophagus, stomach, and duodenum. Endoscopy allows the gastroenterologist to view the patient's upper gastrointestinal tract.

Endotracheal tube: A tube inserted through the mouth or nose and into the windpipe that enables people to breathe during surgery.

Gallbladder: A sac attached to the liver in which bile is stored.

Gastroenterologist: A doctor who specializes in the digestive tract and its diseases.

Graft survival: When a transplanted tissue or organ is accepted by the body and functions properly. The potential for graft survival increases when the recipient and the donor are closely matched, and when immunosuppressive therapy is used.

Hepatic: Having to do with the liver.

Hepatic encephalopathy: See *encephalopathy.*

Hepatitis: A viral infection or non-specific inflammation of the liver that can lead to liver failure. Hepatitis C is the leading cause of liver failure that leads to transplantation.

Hepatologist: A doctor who specializes in the liver and its diseases.

Herpes: A family of viruses that can infect humans and can cause lip sores, genital sores, and shingles.

Human immunodeficiency virus (HIV): A virus that destroys cells in the immune system, which makes it difficult for the body to fight off infections, toxins, poisons, and diseases. HIV causes acquired immune deficiency syndrome (AIDS), a late stage of the viral infection characterized by serious infections, malignancies, and neurologic dysfunctions.

Hypertension: High blood pressure. It can cause damage to the body by over-working the heart and blood vessels.

Immune response: A defensive action by the immune system.

Immune system: The system that protects the body from foreign substances, such as bacteria, viruses, and cancer cells. It can identify a transplanted organ as foreign and try to eliminate the "invader" from the body.

Immunosuppressive agents: Medicines to control the immune system and prevent rejection of a transplanted organ.

Informed consent: A person's voluntary agreement, based on adequate knowledge and understanding of relevant information, to participate in research or to undergo a diagnostic, therapeutic, or preventive procedure.

INR: International normalized ratio; a standardized measure of prothrombin time.

Intravenous: In a vein. Medicines and fluids can be administered through an intravenous line.

Jaundice: Yellowing of the skin and eyes caused by excess bile products in the blood; a common sign of liver disease.

Kidney: One of the two bean-shaped organs located on both sides of the spine, just above the waist. It functions to rid the body of waste and maintain normal amounts of salts, minerals, and fluids through the production of urine.

Liver: The largest internal organ of the body; located in the upper right portion of the abdomen. It performs numerous functions vital to life.

Liver enzymes (SGOT/AST and SGPT/ALT): Substances produced by the liver. When the liver suffers an injury, these enzymes are produced in large amounts and can be measured in the blood.

Living donor: A blood relative or emotionally related friend of the recipient who donates an organ.

Match: The compatibility between a recipient and a donor.

Medicaid: A partnership between the U.S. federal government and the individual states to share the cost of providing medical coverage for recipients of welfare programs. It also allows states to provide the same coverage to low-income workers who are not eli-

gible for welfare. Medicaid programs vary greatly from state to state.

Medicare: The program of the U.S. federal government that provides hospital and medical insurance, through Social Security taxes, to people age 65 and older, those who have permanent kidney failure, and certain people with disabilities.

MELD score: Model of End-Stage Liver Disease score; the calculation used to rank candidates for liver transplantation. Ranges from 6 (not in need) to 40 (urgent need).

MRI: Magnetic resonance imaging. A noninvasive radiologic image obtained using magnetic energy that enables clinicians to see and evaluate internal organs and blood vessels.

Nephrectomy: Surgical removal of the kidney.

Nephrologist: A doctor who specializes in the kidney and its diseases.

Noncompliance: Failure to follow the instructions of one's healthcare providers, such as not taking medicine as prescribed or not showing up for clinic visits.

Oral: By mouth. Many medicines are taken orally in liquid or pill form.

Organ procurement organization (OPO): An organization designated by the Centers for Medicare and Medicaid Services as being responsible for the procurement of organs for transplantation and the promotion of organ donation. OPOs serve as the vital link between the organ donor and the recipient. They are responsible for the identification of donors, and the retrieval, preservation, and transportation of organs for transplantation. They are also involved in data follow-up regarding deceased organ donors. As a resource to the community, OPOs engage in public education on the critical need for organ donation.

Pancreas: A slender organ located below the stomach and above the intestines. It produces insulin and digestive enzymes.

Paracentesis: A procedure to remove ascites (fluid) from the abdomen. After anesthetizing the lower abdomen, a needle is inserted into the fluid and withdrawn, with the fluid often going into suction bottles or bags.

PCP (*Pneumocystis carinii* pneumonia): A type of pneumonia that is most often seen in patients whose immune systems are suppressed (as by immunosuppressive medications).

Potassium: An electrolyte responsible for vital muscle functions.

Prophylaxis: Administration of medication that helps prevent disease.

Prothrombin: A substance produced by the liver that helps with clotting. Prothrombin time is a blood test that indirectly measures the ability of the liver to produce prothrombin; it is also known as the international normalized ratio (INR).

Recipient: The person who receives a donated organ.

Rejection: An attempt by the immune system to destroy a transplanted organ because it recognizes the organ to be a foreign, harmful object.

Renal: Having to do with the kidneys.

Renal failure, acute: When kidneys stop functioning temporarily. Dialysis may be needed until kidney function returns.

Renal failure, chronic: When kidneys slowly lose function over a period of time and do not regain their function. This condition requires long-term dialysis or transplantation.

Sodium: An electrolyte that is the main salt in the blood; also one component of table salt.

Stenosis (stricture): A narrowing of a passage in the body.

Thrush: A fungal infection in the mouth.

Triglycerides: A form of fat that the body makes from sugar, alcohol, and excess calories.

Ultrasound: A noninvasive radiologic image made using sound waves. It enables clinicians to see and evaluate internal organs and blood vessels.

UNOS: United Network for Organ Sharing. The private, nonprofit organization that coordinates the U.S. transplant system through the Department of Health and Human Services' Organ Procurement and Transplantation Network contract.

Uremia: A toxic condition that results from wastes, such as urea and creatinine, accumulating in the blood.

Ureter: A tube that carries urine from the kidney to the bladder.

Urinary tract infection: An infection of one or more parts of the urinary tract.

Varices (esophageal): Enlarged and swollen veins at the bottom of the esophagus, near the stomach. This condition is often caused by increased pressure in the liver, and can cause these veins to bleed.

Ventilator: A machine that helps a person breathe.

Virus: A very small germ that causes infection.

Xenotransplantation: Transplantation of an animal organ into a human. Although xenotransplantation is highly experimental, many scientists view it as an eventual solution to the shortage of human organs.

Index

A

Abdominal surgery, risk of, 52–53
ABO typing, 59–60, 183
Acetaminophen (Tylenol), 70–71, 105–106, 135
Acifex (rabeprazole), 146
Activity level after transplantation, 111–112
Acute rejection, 152–153
Acute renal failure, 11, 187
Acyclovir (Zovirax), 144
Adalat (nifedipine), 146
AFP (alphafetoprotein) blood test, 33
Age, and risk of renal failure, 159
Alanine aminotransferase (ALT), 155, 183
Albumin, 52, 183
Alcohol use
    abstaining from after transplantation, 106, 108–109
    cirrhosis and, 3, 4, 5t
    qualifying for transplantation, 32–33
Alcoholic liver disease, 96
Aldactone (spironolactone), 148
Allocation of organs. *See* Organ allocation
Allograft, 154, 183
Allopurinol (Zyloprim), 133
Alpha-1 antitrypsin deficiency, 4, 96
Alphafetoprotein (AFP) blood test, 33
ALT, 155, 183
American Liver Foundation, 31, 179
American Organ Transplant Association, 179
Amoxicillin, 116
Anatomy of the liver, 162–163, 162f, 163f
Androstenedione, 74
Anesthesia, 80, 183
Antacid
    defined, 183
    interactions with immunosuppressants, 132
Anti-infection drugs. *See* Antibacterials

Anti-inflammatory drugs, 131–132
Anti-rejection drugs. *See* Immunosuppressive agents
Antibacterials, 139–140
    ciprofloxacin (Cipro), 140
    infection, 153
    levofloxacin (levaquin), 140
    trimethoprim-sulfamethoxazole (TMP-SMZ, Bactrim, Cotrim, Septra), 139–140
Antibiotics. *See* Antibacterials
Antibody, 99, 183
Antifungal medications, 141–143
    clotrimazole (Mycelex), 141–142
    fluconazole (Diflucan), 143
    ketoconazole (Nizoral), 142–143
    mycostatin (Nystatin), 141
Antihypertensive medications, 146–147
Antiproliferative medications, 132
Antiviral medications, 143–144
    acyclovir (Zovirax), 144
    ganciclovir (Cytovene), 143–144
    for infection, 153
    valganciclovir (Valcyte), 143–144
Appetite, after transplantation, 119
Aristolochic acid, 73
Ascites, 9–10, 14, 67, 69
    defined, 5, 183
    in HRS, 42
Aspartate aminotransferase (AST), 155, 183
AST, 155, 183
Atenolol (Tenormin), 146
Atorvastatin (Lipitor), 149
Autoimmune hepatitis, 96
Autoimmune liver disease, recurrence, 96–97
Availability of organs, 13
Axid (nizatidine), 145
Azathioprine (Imuran), 133–134
Azithromycin (Zithromax), 116

B

Bacteria
    defined, 3, 183
    infection caused by, 15
Bactrim (trimethoprim-sulfamethoxazole), 139–140
Basiliximab (Simulect), 135–136
Benadryl, 135
Biaxin (clarithromycin), 116
Bile, 2, 183
Bile duct
    complications after surgery, 92
    damage to, retransplantation and, 113
    reconstruction of, 83, 83f
Bile leak, 92, 183
Bile tube, 83, 87–88, 183
Biliary stenosis, 92, 184
Bilirubin, 11, 49, 62, 184
Biopsy
    defined, 184
    liver (*See* Liver biopsy)
Birth control, after transplantation, 117
Bitter orange, 74
Bladder, 15, 43, 184
Bleeding
    complications after surgery, 93
    variceal, 8, 14
Blood clot, after surgery, 93
Blood flow to the liver, 6–8, 7f
Blood pressure. *See* Hypertension; Hypotension
Blood type matches, acceptable, 59–61, 60t
Blood type O liver, 51, 60–61
Blood urea nitrogen (BUN), 42, 184
BMI (body mass index), 38
Brain death, 25, 26, 184
Breathing tube, 80–81, 85–86
Bumetamide (Bumex), 148
Bumex (bumetamide), 148
BUN (blood urea nitrogen), 42, 184

C

Cadaver, defined, 25, 184
Cadaver liver, 24–26
    defined, 24–25
    eligibility to be a donor, 26
    and living donor transplantation, compared, 164, 173–174
    number of transplants performed (2004-2005), 25
    organ donors, 25

single donor, for liver-kidney transplantation, 45
split donor liver transplantation, 165
Cadaveric donor, 184
Calcineurin inhibitors, 129, 130
Cancer
    of the liver, and qualifying for a transplant, 33–35, 75–76
    skin, 116
Candidates for transplantation, 13–14, 20–21
Capillaries
    hepatic vein, 7
    portal, 7
Capoten (captopril), 146
Captopril (Capoten), 146
Carbohydrates in the diet, 119–120
Cardiac, 184
Cardiac death, 25
Cardiologist, 39, 184
Cardizem (diltiazem), 146
Caregiving team, experience of, 22
Cartia (diltiazem), 146
Celexa, 72
CellCept (mycophenolate mofetil), 117, 118, 125, 132–133, 159
Centers for Medicare and Medicaid Services, 37, 56, 179
Chaparral, 74
Chemotherapy, tumor recurrence rates and, 34
Child-Turcotte-Pugh score, 52–53
Children's Liver Association for Support Services, 179
Choledochocholedochostomy, 83, 83f
Choledochojejunostomy, 83, 83f
Cholestatic liver disease, vitamin supplementation and, 68
Cholesterol, 67, 184
Cholesterol-lowering agents, 71–72, 148–149
Chronic rejection (CR), 110, 113, 154, 184
Chronic renal failure, 158–159, 187
Cimetidine (Tagamet), 142, 145
Cipro (ciproflxacin), 140
Ciprofloxacin (Cipro), 140
Cirrhosis, 4, 5t
    blood flow, 7
    causes, 3, 4, 5t
    compensated, 5, 12
    complications, 5–6, 13, 14t
    confusion and sleepiness with, 10–11
    decompensated, 5, 12
    defined, 2, 3, 184

hepatic, recurrence of HCV disease, 97–100
kidney failure and, 44
need for a transplant, 13–14
signs and symptoms, 4
Clarithromycin (Biaxin), 116
Cleosin (clindamycin), 116
Clindamycin (Cleosin), 116
Clotrimazole (Mycelex), 141–142
CMV (cytomegalovirus), 113, 138–139, 184
Cocaine, abstaining from after transplantation, 106
Comfrey, 74
Commitment from friends and family, 29–30
Compensated cirrhosis, 5, 12
Complications after transplantation, 13, 151–159
    bile duct, 92
    bleeding, 93
    chronic renal failure, 158–159
    effects of long-term immunosuppression, 156–158
    infection, 91–92, 153
    liver biopsy, 154–156
    primary graft nonfunction, 91
    rejection, 89–91
        acute, 152–153
        chronic, 154
    renal dysfunction, 92
    thrombosis (blood clot), 93
    vascular, 92–93
Computerized tomography (CT) scan, 33, 184
Conception after transplantation, 125, 133
Cotrim (trimethoprim-sulfamethoxazole), 139–140
Creatinine, 15, 42, 184
Criteria, medical, 28, 184
CT scan, 33, 184
Cyclosporine (Neoral, Sandimmune, Gengraf, Eon), 116–117, 129–130, 137, 157, 158, 159
Cytomegalovirus (CMV), 138–139, 184
    retransplantation and, 113
Cytovene (ganciclovir), 143–144

D

Daclizumab (Zenapax), 136
Daily record, 106
Darvocet (propoxyphene), 70
DCD (donation after cardiac death), 27
Death, after transplantation, 109–111

Decompensated cirrhosis, 5, 12
Deltasone (prednisone), 131–132
Demadex (torsemide), 148
Dental hygiene, 116–117
Dental work, medications before, 116–117
Department of Public Health, 179
Diabetes, 38, 157, 184
Dialysis, 158–159, 184
    for HRS, 42
    before transplantation, 17
Diets
    after transplantation, 118–120
    for people with liver disease, 67–68
Diflucan (fluconazole), 143
Digestive system, protective medications, 145–146
    histamine-2 (H$_2$) acid blockers, 145
    proton pump inhibitors, 145–146
Dilacor (diltiazem), 146
Diltiazem (Cardizem, Cardia, Dilacor, Tiazac), 146
Dirithromycin (Dynabac), 116
Diseases, cured by transplantation, 95
Diuretics, 148
    side effects, 158
Doctors. *See* Physicians
Domino liver transplantation, 28–29
Donation after cardiac death (DCD), 27
Donor. *See also* Living donor liver transplantation (LDLT)
    cadaver liver, 26
    defined, 25, 184
    donation after cardiac death (DCD), 27
    extended criteria donor (ECD), 27–28
    historical information about, 57–58
    ideal donor, 27–28
    increasing the donor pool, 176–177
    living donor defined, 26
    meeting the family of, 123–124
    sex of, 59
Driving after transplantation, 120–121
Dynabac, 116
Dynabac (dirithromycin), 116

E

Edema, 67, 184
Electrocardiogram, 40, 184
Electrocardiogram leads, 87
Electrolyte, 11, 184–185
Eligibility to be a donor, cadaver liver, 26
Enalapril (Vasotec), 146
Encephalopathy

defined, 185
hepatic (HE), 6
End-stage liver disease, 12
  living donor transplantation for, 164, 165
  MELD score, 14, 15
Endoscope, 8
Endoscopy, 8–9, 185
Endotracheal tube, 185
  insertion, 80–81
  removal, 85–86
Eon (cyclosporine), 116–117, 129–130, 137, 159
Epstein-Barr virus infection, 158
Erythromycin, 116
Esomeprozole (Nexium), 146
Esophageal varices, 5
Esophagus, evaluation of, 9
Evaluation, transplantation, 39–41
Exercise, after transplantation, 111–112
Extended criteria donor (ECD), 27–28

F

Familial amyloidotic polyneuropathy (FAP), 16
  domino liver transplantation, 28–29
Family of the donor, meeting with, 123–124
Famotidine (Pepcid), 142, 145
Fatigue, after transplantation, 121–122
Fats in the diet, 120
Fatty liver disease, 96
FHF (fulminant hepatic failure), 16, 54–55
Fibrosing cholestatic hepatitis, 98
Fibrosis, 12
Financial coordinator, 35, 40
Five-year mortality, 110
FK-506 (tacrolimus), 130–131, 137, 159
Florinef (fludrocortisone), 147
Fluconazole (Diflucan), 143
Fludrocortisone (Florinef), 147
Fluid retention, 67
Foley catheter
  insertion, 81
  removal, 87
Follow-up visits, 104–105
Fulminant hepatic failure (FHF), 16, 54–55
Furosemide (Lasix), 148

G

Gallbladder, 2, 185
Ganciclovir (Cytovene), 143–144
Gastroenterologist, 8, 9, 185

Gastroesophageal reflux disease (GERD), 145–146
Gender, and risk of renal failure, 159
Gengraf (cyclosporine), 116–117, 129–130, 137, 159
GERD (gastroesophageal reflux disease), 145–146
Germander, 74
Glutathione production, 71
Graft survival
  defined, 22, 185
  statistics, 21

H

HCTZ (hydrochlorothiazide), 148
Healthcare professionals, transplant evaluation, 40–41
Healthcare proxy, 65
Hepatic, 2, 185
Hepatic artery thrombosis, retransplantation and, 113
Hepatic cirrhosis
  recurrence of HBV disease after transplantation, 101
  recurrence of HCV disease after transplantation, 97–100
Hepatic encephalopathy (HE), 6, 10–11, 14
  diet considerations, 68
  TIPS procedure, 68–69
  treatment, 11
Hepatitis
  autoimmune, 96
  defined, 4, 185
Hepatitis A virus (HAV), 16
Hepatitis B immune globulin (HBIg), treatment after transplantation, 101
Hepatitis B virus (HBV), 4, 16
  recurrence of after transplantation, 101
  testing donor organs for, 57
Hepatitis C virus (HCV), 4, 100
  recurrence of after transplantation, 97–98
  retransplantation and, 113, 114
  treatment, 98–100
  testing donor organs for, 57
Hepatologist, 10, 185
Hepatorenal syndrome (HRS), 41–42
Herbal medications, 72–75
Hereditary hemochromatosis, 4
Heroin, abstaining from after transplantation, 106
Herpes, 112, 185
Histamine-2 (H$_2$) acid blockers, 145

HIV
   See Human immunodeficiency virus (HIV)
Hospital
   discharge, 104
   length of stay after surgery, 88–89
   time needed to get to after notification,
      76–77
   what to bring, 64
HRS (hepatorenal syndrome), 41–42
Human immunodeficiency virus (HIV)
   defined, 21, 185
   HIV-positive status, 20
   testing donor organs for, 57
Hydrochlorothiazide (HCTZ), 148
Hydromorphone (Vicodin), 70
Hypertension, 119
   defined, 185
   incidence, 157
   medications, 146–147
   portal, 6–8
Hypotension medications, 147

I

Ideal donor, 27–28
Immune response, 154, 185
Immune system, 11, 185
Immunosuppressive agents, 15, 91, 125,
      127–150, 136–138
   acute rejection, 152–153
   administration of, 128
   complications, 156–158
   defined, 128–129, 185
   drugs and their side effects
      azathioprine (Imuran), 133–134
      basiliximab (Simulect), 135–136
      cyclosporine (Neoral, Sandimmune,
         GenGraf, Eon), 129–130
      daclizumab (Zenapax), 136
      muromonab-CD-3 (OKT3), 135
      mycophenolate mofetil (CellCept,
         Myfortin), 132–133
      prednisone (Deltasone, Orasone),
         131–132
      sirolumus (Rapamune, Rapamycin), 134
      tacrolimus (Prograf, FK-506), 130–131
   need for, 128
   patient survival, 137
   stopping pre-transplant drugs, 138–139
   stopping treatment, 128, 136–138
Imuran (azathioprine), 133–134
Incision, surgery, 81
Infection, after transplantation, 91–92, 153

Infectious disease, testing donor organs for,
      57–58
Infectious disease doctor, 40
Informed consent, 123, 185
INR. *See* International normalized ratio (INR)
Intensive care unit (ICU), 84
Interactions, drug, 132, 149–150. *See also*
      specific drugs
Interferon/ribavirin combination therapy,
      recurrent HCV disease, 99–100
International normalized ratio (INR), 15,
      49, 62
   defined, 2, 186
Intrahepatic, 69
Intravenous, 8, 186
Intravenous lines, 86–87

J

Jackson-Pratt drains
   insertion, 83–84
   removal, 87
Jaundice, 4, 5, 14, 186

K

Kava, 74
Ketoconazole (Nizoral), 142–143
Kidney
   defined, 15, 186
   function of, 43–44
Kidney failure, 42
   with cirrhosis, 44
Kidney function, pre-transplantation, 159
Kidney-liver transplantation, 17, 43–45
   rejection of kidney, 44–45

L

Lansoprazole (Prevacid), 146
Lasix (furosemide), 148
Latino Organization for Liver Awareness
      (LOLA), 180
LDLT. *See* Living donor liver transplan-
      tation (LDLT)
Length of hospital stay after surgery, 88–89
Levaquin (levofloxacin), 140
Levofloxacin (Levaquin), 140
Lipitor (atorvastatin), 149
Lisinopril (Zestril), 146
Liver
   anatomy, 162–163, 162f, 163f
   cadaver liver, 24–26
   cancer of, 33–35, 75–76

Index

defined, 186
description of, 2
end-stage liver disease, 12, 14, 15
failure after transplantation, 113
function, determining, 11–12, 152
function of, 2
importance of, 2
location in the abdomen, 3f
regeneration, 109
Liver allograft, 154
Liver biopsy, 12, 90, 152, 154–156
complications, 156
procedure, 90f, 156
staging, 155
Liver enzymes, 72, 155, 186
Liver-kidney transplantation, 43–45
rejection of kidney, 44–45
Living donor liver transplantation
(LDLT), 161–178
anatomy of the liver, 162–163, 162f, 163f
and cadaver liver transplantation, compared, 164, 173–174
defined, 163–164
donors
benefits to, 168–169
evaluation process, 169–170
going back to work, 172–173
hospital stay, 172–173
immediate benefits to, 166
living donor defined, 26, 186
negative psychological consequences
to, 168
potential, 60t, 166–167
rejection of, 175–176
risks, 167, 172
who pays for the donor, 170–171, 173
the future for, 176–177
liver donated by relative, immunosuppressive agents and, 174–175
need for, 165–166
resources for learning about, 177–181
split donor transplant, 165
surgery, 170–171
Lobelia, 75
LOLA (Latino Organization for Liver
Awareness), 180
Lopressor (metoprolol), 146
Lovastatin (Mevacor), 149
Lymphoma, transplant-associated, 158

M

Magnetic resonance imaging (MRI), 33, 186
Marijuana, abstaining from after transplantation, 106
Match, 26, 186
Medicaid, 37, 186
Medical evaluation tests, 39–40
Medicare, 37, 180, 186
Medications. See also specific names
anti-infection, 139–140
anti-rejection (See Immunosuppressive
agents)
antibacterials, 139–140
antifungal, 141–143
antihypertensive, 146–147
antiproliferative, 132
antiviral, 143–144
cholesterol-lowering agents, 71–72,
148–149
before dental work, 116–117
diuretics, 148
following transplantation, 105–106
hepatitis B immune globulin (HBIg), 101
interactions, 149–150
interferon/ribavirin combination therapy,
99–100
noncompliance with, 20
nontraditional, 72–75
oral, to control hepatitis B, 101
for pain, 70–71
to protect the digestive system, 145–146
psychiatric medications, 72
side effects, 13, 129–135
MELD scores, 26, 44, 45, 48–50, 49t, 54, 56
calculating, 49
defined, 186
end-stage renal disease, 14, 15
and mortality equivalents, 49–50, 49t
patients with liver cancer, 75–76
prioritizing of patients by, 50–52
TIPS procedure and, 69
waiting time and, 61–62
Men, special health issues for, 118
Metoprolol (Lopressor), 146
Mevacor (lovastatin), 149
Milan Criteria, 33–34, 34f
Model of End-Stage Liver Disease
(MELD) score. See MELD scores
Mortality, after transplantation, 109–111
MRI (magnetic resonance imaging), 33, 186
Muromonab-CD3 (OKT3), 135
Mycelex (clotrimazole), 141–142

Mycophenolate mofetil (CellCept), mycophenolate sodium (Myfortic), 117, 118, 125, 132–133, 159
Mycostatin (nystatin), 141
Myfortic (mycophenolate mofetil), 117, 118, 125, 132–133, 159

N

Nasogastric tube
    insertion, 81
    removal, 86
National Council on Patient Information and Education (NCPIE), 180
National Digestive Diseases Information Clearinghouse, 180
National Foundation for Transplants, 180
National Institutes of Health, 180
Neoral (cyclosporine), 116–117, 129–130, 137, 159
Nephrectomy, 186
Nephrologist, 39, 186
Nexium (esomeprozole), 146
Nifedipine (Procardia, Adalat), 146
Nizatidine (Axid), 145
Nizoral (ketoconazole), 142–143
Non-African Americans, risk of renal failure, 159
Non-alcoholic steatohepatitis, 96
Non-Caucasians, risk of renal failure, 159
Noncompliance with providers' instruction, 20, 21, 186
Nontraditional medications, 72–75
    definitely hazardous, 73
    likely hazardous, 74–75
    very likely hazardous, 73–74
Nutritionist, 40
Nystatin (mycostatin), 141

O

Obesity, 157
OKT3 (muromonab), 135
Omeprazole (Prilosec), 145–146
One-year mortality, 110
Operative mortality, 109–110
OPO. *See* Organ procurement organization (OPO)
Oral, 70, 186
Orasone (prednisone), 131–132
Organ allocation, 13, 47–62
    being unavailable for, 55
    blood types, acceptable, 59–61, 60t
    Child's score, 52–53
    listings at more than one center, 58–59
    MELD score, 48–50, 50–52, 61–62

organ distribution by region, 55–56
    organizations, 48
    sex of donors, 59
    Status 1 patients, 54–56
    testing of donor organs, 57–58
    waiting list, 50–52, 52f
        moving up or down on, 53–54
        national list, 53
    waiting time, 61–62
Organ/glandular extracts, 74–75
Organ Procurement and Transportation Network (OPTN), 48, 56
Organ procurement organization (OPO), 48, 56, 186–187
    privacy policies, 124
Organizations, addresses and websites, 179–181
Orthoclone OKT3 (muromonab), 135
    lymphoma and, 158
Overlap syndrome, recurrence of after transplantation, 96
Oxycodone (Percocet), 70

P

Pain medications, 70–71
Pancreas, 16, 187
Pantoprazole (Protonix), 146
Pap smear, 158
Paracentesis, 10, 187
Patient survival statistics, 21
Paxil, 72
Paying for the transplant, 35–37
    costs of, 35–36
    financial coordinator, 35
    insurance coverage, 35–36
    living donor, 170–171, 173
    no insurance coverage, 36
    professional help for, 35
    social worker, 35
PCP (*pneumocystis carinii* pneumonia), 138, 139
    defined, 187
    prevention, 139
Pennyroyal oil, 75
Pepcid (famotidine), 142, 145
Percocet (oxycodone), 70
Physical preparation for the transplantation, 66
Physicians
    infectious disease, 40
    post-surgery, 115–117
    transplant surgeon, 40

Piggyback technique, 82
Pneumocystis carinii pneumonia (PCP), 138, 139
    defined, 187
    prevention, 139
Polycystic liver disease, 16–17
Portal capillaries, 7
Portal hypertension, 6–8
    TIPS procedure, 68–70
Portosystemic, 69
Post-transplant lymphoproliferative disease (PTLD), 158
Potassium, 131, 187
Pravachol (pravastatin), 149
Pravastatin (Pravachol), 149
Prednisone (Deltasone, Orasone), 119, 131–132, 137
Pregnancy
    after transplantation, 117, 125, 133
    medications to avoid during, 133, 140–141, 144, 149
Preparing for transplantation, 63–77
    amount of time to get to the hospital, 76–77
    establish a heathcare proxy, 65
    how to prepare for the call, 64–66
    patients with liver cancer, 75–76
    preparing yourself physically, 66–67
    special diets for people with liver disease, 67–68
    TIPS procedure, 68–70
    use of cholesterol-lowering agents, 71–72
    use of nontraditional medications, 72–75
    use of pain medications, 70–71
    use of psychiatric medications, 72
    what to bring to the hospital, 64
Prevacid (lansoprazole), 146
Prilosec (omeprazole), 145–146
Primary biliary cirrhosis, 4
    recurrence of after transplantation, 96
    vitamin supplementation and, 68
Primary graft nonfunction (PGNF), 54, 55
    after surgery, 91
    retransplantation and, 112–113
Primary sclerosing cholangitis, 4
    recurrence of after transplantation, 96
    vitamin supplementation and, 68
Privacy policies, donors and recipients, 123–124
Procardia (nifedipine), 146
Prograf (tacrolimus), 130–131, 137, 159
Program for transplantation
    choosing the right one, 21–23

caregiving team, experience of, 22
    proximity to the transplant center, 22
    statistics, 21–22
    coordination of care, 22–23
Progressive liver disease, after transplantation, 113–114
Prophylaxis
    defined, 187
    against hepatitis C virus after transplantation, 99
Propoxyphene (Darvocet), 70
Protein in the diet
    after transplantation, 119
    restriction, 68
Prothrombin, 187
    defined, 2
Proton pump inhibitors, 145–146
Protonix (pantoprazole), 146
Prozac, 72
Psychiatric medications, 72
Psychiatrist, 40
PTLD (post-transplant lymphoproliferative disease), 158

Q
Qualifying for a transplant
    alcohol abuse and, 32–33
    liver cancer and, 33–35, 75–76
Questions to ask the transplant team, 23–24

R
Rabeprazole (Aciphex), 146
Ranitidine (Zantac), 142, 145
Rapamune (sirolimus), 134, 137, 159
Rapamycin (sirolimus), 134, 137, 159
Recipient
    commitment to aftercare, 21
    defined, 21, 187
Record, daily, 106
Recurrent liver disease, 95–101
    diseases cured by transplantation, 95
    fibrosing cholestatic hepatitis, 98
    hepatitis B virus (HBV) disease, 101
    hepatitis C virus (HCV) disease, 97–98
    treatment, 98–100
    retransplantation and, 113
    risk of recurrence of autoimmune diseases, 95–96
Regeneration of the liver, 109
Regional procurement of organs, United States, 51–52, 52f
Rejection, 89–91

acute, 152–153
chronic, 110, 154
    retransplantation and, 113
defined, 45, 187
of kidney, in liver-kidney transplantation,
    44–45
Renal, 187
Renal dysfunction, after surgery, 92
Renal failure, 11
acute, 11, 187
chronic, 158–159, 187
Research studies, 177
participation in, 122–123
Resources, 179–181
Responsibilities, regarding medications,
    105–106
Rest, after transplant, 112
Rh factor, 60

S

Salt in the diet
    after transplantation, 120
    restriction, 9
Sandimmune (cyclosporine), 116–117,
    129–130, 137, 159
Scarring of the liver, 2–3
Scientific Registry of Transplant Recipients,
    180
Scullcap, 75
Selective serotonin reuptake inhibitors
    (SSRIs), 72
Sepsis, 15–16
Septra (trimethoprim-sulfamethoxazole),
    139–140
Sex of donors, 59
Sexual activity, after transplantation, 112
SGOT/AST, 186
SGPT/ALT, 186
Shunt, 69
Side effects, immunosuppressive agents. See
    Specific medications
Simulect (basiliximab), 135–136
Simvastatin (Zocor), 149
Single donor, for liver-kidney transplanta-
    tion, 45
Sirolumus (Rapamune, Rapamycin), 134,
    137, 159
Skin cancer, 116
Social Security Disability Insurance, 37
Social worker, 35, 40
Sodium in the diet, 146
    after transplantation, 120

restriction, 9
    sodium defined, 187
Spironolactone (Aldactone), 148
Split donor transplantation, 165
SSRIs (selective serotonin reuptake
    inhibitors), 72
Staging, liver biopsy, 155
Status 1 patients, organ allocation, 54–56
Stenosis, 92, 187
Support groups, 30–31
Surgery, 79–94. See also Transplantation
    anesthesia, 80
    becoming fully independent again, 93–94
    bile tube, 83, 87–88
    complications
        bile duct, 92
        bleeding, 93
        infection, 91–92
        primary graft nonfunction, 91
        rate of post-surgery, 13
        rejection, 89–91
        renal dysfunction, 92
        thrombosis (blood clot), 93
        vascular, 92–93
    doctors who will care for you post-sur-
        gery, 115–117
    electrocardiogram leads, 87
    endotracheal tube
        insertion, 80–81
        removal, 85–86
    Foley catheter
        insertion, 81
        removal, 87
    incision, 81
    intravenous lines, 86–87
    Jackson-Pratt drains
        placed in the abdomen, 83–84
        removal, 87
    length of hospital stay, 88–89
    length of the operation, 80–84
    living donor liver transplantation, 170–171
    nasogastric tube
        insertion, 81
        removal, 86
    piggyback technique, 82
    reconstruction of the bile ducts, 83, 83f
    restrictions after, 114–115
    venovenous bypass, 82, 82f
    waking up from, 84–85

T

Tacrolimus (Prograf, FK-506), 130–131, 137, 158, 159
Tagamet (cimetidine), 142, 145
Ten-year mortality, 110
Tenormin (atenolol), 146
Testing of donor organs, 57–58
Three-year mortality, 110
Thrombosis (blood clot), after surgery, 93
Thrush, 141, 187
Tiazac (diltiazem), 146
Time needed to get to the hospital after notification, 76–77
TIPS, 68–70
   contraindications for, 69–70
   procedure, 69
   reasons for, 68–69
TMP-SMZ (trimethoprim-sulfamethoxazole), 139–140
Torsemide (Demadex), 148
Transjugular, 69
Transjugular Intrahepatic Portosystemic Shunt (TIPS), 69–70
Transplant-associated lymphoma, 158
Transplant evaluation, 39–41
Transplant Foundation, 180
Transplant nurse coordinator, 40–41
Transplant Recipients International Organization (TRIO), 181
Transplant surgeon, 40
Transplant team, when to call, 107–108
Transplantation. *See also* Preparing for transplantation; Surgery
   being too sick for, 14–16
   candidates for, 13–14, 20–21
   choosing the right program, 21–23
   conditions that warrant transplantation, 16–17
   domino liver transplantation, 28–29
   how long will the liver last, 109–111
   liver-kidney, 43–45
   second or third transplants, 112–114
Transthyretin, 16
Travel after transplantation, 112
Triglycerides, 134, 187
Trimethoprim-sulfamethoxazole (TMP-SMZ, Bactrim, Cotrim, Septra), 139–140
Tylenol (acetaminophen), 70–71, 105–106, 135

U

Ultrasound, 33, 187
United Network for Organ Sharing (UNOS), 21–22, 22, 48
   address and website, 181
   defined, 187
   regions of the United States, 51–52, 52f, 55, 62
   waiting list, 166–167
United Organization for Organ Sharing, 115
Upper abdomen, 81f
Uremia, 44, 187
Ureter, 43, 188
Urethra, 43
Urinary tract infection
   defined, 188
   treatment, 140
Urine, 43
U.S. Department of Human Services, 48

V

Valcyte (valganciclovir), 143–144
Valganciclovir (Valcyte), 143–144
Variceal bleeding, 8, 14
   TIPS procedure and, 69
Varices, esophageal, 5, 188
Vascular complications after surgery, 92–93
Vasotec (enalapril), 146
Venovenous bypass, 82, 82f
Ventilator, 25, 188
Vicodin (hydromorphone), 70
Virus, 4, 188
Vitamin supplementation, 68

W

Waiting list, organ allocation, 50–52, 52f
   moving up or down on, 53–54
   national list, 53
Waiting time, organ allocation, 61–62
Waking up from surgery, 84–85
Weight gain, after transplantation, 119
Weight limit for recipients, 38–39
Wilson's disease, 16, 96
Women, special health issues for, 117–118
   pregnancy
      after transplantation, 117, 125, 133

medications to avoid during, 133,
140–141, 144, 149

X

Xenotransplantation, 177, 188

Y

Yohimbe, 75

Z

Zantac (ranitidine), 142, 145
Zenapax (daclizumab), 136
Zestril (lisinopril), 146
Zithromax (azithromycin), 116
Zocor (simvistatin), 149
Zovirax (acyclovir), 144
Zyloprim (allopurinol), 133

Index